Transplantation at a Glance

Menna Clatworthy

University Lecturer in Renal Medicine
University of Cambridge
Cambridge, UK

Christopher Watson

Professor of Transplantation
University of Cambridge
Cambridge, UK

Michael Allison

Consultant Hepatologist
Addenbrooke's Hospital
Cambridge, UK

John Dark

Professor of Cardiothoracic Surgery
The Freeman Hospital
Newcastle-upon-Tyne, UK

T0252663

WILEY-BLACKWELL

A John Wiley & Sons, Ltd., Publication

Registered office: John Wiley & Sons, Ltd, The Atrium, Southern Gate, Chichester, West Sussex, PO19 8SQ, UK

Editorial offices: 9600 Garsington Road, Oxford, OX4 2DQ, UK
   The Atrium, Southern Gate, Chichester, West Sussex, PO19 8SQ, UK
   111 River Street, Hoboken, NJ 07030-5774, USA

For details of our global editorial offices, for customer services and for information about how to apply for permission to reuse the copyright material in this book please see our website at www.wiley.com/wiley-blackwell.

Library of Congress Cataloging-in-Publication Data
Transplantation at a glance / Menna Clatworthy . . . [et al.].
   p. ; cm. – (At a glance)
Includes bibliographical references and index.
ISBN 978-0-470-65842-0 (pbk. : alk. paper)
I. Clatworthy, Menna.   II. Series: At a glance series (Oxford, England).
[DNLM: 1. Organ Transplantation.   2. Transplantation Immunology.   3. Transplants. WO 660]
  617.9'54–dc23

Set in 9/11.5 pt Times by Toppan Best-set Premedia Limited

1   2012

Contents

Preface

The early attempts at transplantation in the first half of the 20th century were limited by technical challenges and ignorance of the immune response. Half a century later, with an appreciation of some aspects of human immunology, the first successful renal transplant was performed between identical twins. From these beginnings transplantation has progressed from being an experimental treatment available to a few, to a thriving discipline providing life-changing treatment for many. Its power to dramatically transform the quality and quantity of life continues to capture and inspire those involved at all levels of care. Transplantation is a truly multidisciplinary specialty where input from physicians, surgeons, tissue-typists, nurses, coordinators and many others is required in the provision of optimal care. It is also a rapidly moving discipline in which advances in surgical technique and immunological knowledge are constantly being used to improve outcomes. As a newcomer to the field, the breadth of knowledge required can appear bewildering, and it is with this in mind that we have written *Transplantation at a Glance*. We hope that in this short, illustrated text we have provided the reader with a succinct, yet comprehensive overview of the most important aspects of transplantation. The book is designed to be easily read and to rapidly illuminate this exciting subject. We have long felt that many aspects of transplantation are best conveyed by diagrammatic or pictorial representation, and it was this conviction that led to the creation of *Transplantation at a Glance*. In particular, the two fundamentals of transplantation, basic immunology and surgical technique, are best learned through pictures. For those approaching transplantation without a significant background in immunology or the manifestations of organ failure, we have provided an up-to-date, crash course that allows the understanding of concepts important in transplantation so that subsequent chapters can be easily mastered. For those without a surgical background, the essential operative principles are simply summarised. Most importantly, throughout the text we have aimed to provide a practical and clinically relevant guide to transplantation which we hope will assist those wishing to rapidly familiarise themselves with the field, regardless of background knowledge.

MRC
CJEW

List of abbreviations

6-MP	6-mercaptopurine
ACR	acute cellular rejection; albumin–creatinine ratio
ADCC	antibody-dependent cellular cytotoxicity
ADH	antidiuretic hormone
AKI	acute kidney injury
ALD	alcohol-related liver disease
ALG	anti-lymphocyte globulin
ALP	alkaline phosphatase
ALT	alanine transaminase
AMR	antibody-mediated rejection
ANCA	antineutrophil cytoplasmic antibody
APC	antigen-presenting cell
APD	automated peritoneal dialysis
APKD	adult polycystic kidney disease
ARB	angiotensin receptor blocker
AST	aspartate transaminase
ATG	anti-thymocyte globulin
ATN	acute tubular necrosis
AV	atrioventricular
AVF	arteriovenous fistula
BAL	bronchoalveolar lavage
BCR	B cell receptor
BMI	body mass index
BOS	bronchiolitis obliterans syndrome
BP	blood pressure
CABG	coronary artery bypass graft
CAPD	continuous ambulatory peritoneal dialysis
CAV	cardiac allograft vasculopathy
CD	cluster of differentiation
CDC	complement-dependent cytotoxicity
CDR	complementarity-determining region
CF	cystic fibrosis
CKD	chronic kidney disease
CMV	cytomegalovirus
CNI	calcineurin inhibitor
CO	carbon monoxide; cardiac output
COPD	chronic obstructive pulmonary disease
CPET	cardiopulmonary exercise testing
CPP	cerebral perfusion pressure
cRF	calculated reaction frequency
CRP	C-reactive protein
CSF	cerebrospinal fluid
CT	computed tomography
CTA	composite tissue allotransplantation
CXR	chest X-ray
DAMP	danger/damage-associated molecular pattern
DBD	donation after brain death
DC	dendritic cell
DCD	donation after circulatory death
DGF	delayed graft function
DLCO	diffusing capacity of the lung for carbon monoxide
DSA	donor-specific antibodies
DTT	dithiothreitol
EBV	Epstein-Barr virus
ECG	electrocardiogram
ECMO	extra-corporeal membrane oxygenator
EEG	electroencephalogram
ELISA	enzyme-linked immunosorbent assay
EPO	erythropoietin
EPS	encapsulating peritoneal sclerosis
ERCP	endoscopic retrograde cholangio-pancreatography
ESRF	end-stage renal failure
EVLP	ex vivo lung perfusion
FcγR	Fc-gamma receptor
FEV$_1$	forced expiratory volume in 1 second
FFP	fresh frozen plasma
FGF	fibroblast growth factor
FP	fusion protein
FSGS	focal segmental glomerulosclerosis
FVC	forced vital capacity
GDM	gestational diabetes mellitus
GERD	gastro-oesophageal reflux disease
GFR	glomerular filtration rate
GN	glomerulonephritis
HAI	healthcare-associated infection
HAS	human albumin solution
HBIG	hepatitis B immune globulin
HBV	hepatitis B virus
HCV	hepatitis C virus
HD	haemodialysis
HLA	human leucocyte antigen
HSP	heat shock protein
HSV	herpes simplex virus
IAK	islet after kidney
ICP	intracranial pressure
IF	interstitial fibrosis
IFALD	intestinal failure-associated liver disease
IFN	interferon
IL	interleukin
IMPDH	inosine monophosphate dehydrogenase
IMV	inferior mesenteric vein
INR	international normalised ratio
IPF	idiopathic pulmonary fibrosis
ITA	islet transplantation alone
ITU	intensive therapy unit
IVC	inferior vena cava
JVP	jugular venous pressure
KIR	killer-cell immunoglobulin-like receptor
KS	Kaposi's sarcoma
LV	left ventricular
LVAD	left ventricular assist device
LVEDP	left ventricular end diastolic pressure
LVH	left ventricular hypertrophy
mAb	monoclonal antibody
MAC	membrane attack complex
MAP	mean arterial pressure
MELD	model for end-stage liver disease
MHC	major histocompatibility complex
MI	myocardial infarction
MMF	mycophenolate mofetil

MODY	maturity onset diabetes of the young	**RFA**	radiofrequency ablation
MPA	mycophenolic acid	**RRT**	renal replacement therapy
MPAP	mean pulmonary arterial pressure	**SAP**	serum amyloid protein
MPS	mycophenolate sodium	**SMA**	superior mesenteric artery
MR	magnetic resonance	**SMV**	superior mesenteric vein
MRSA	methicillin-resistant *Staphylococcus aureus*	**SPK**	simultaneous pancreas and kidney
NAFLD	non-alcoholic fatty liver disease	**T3**	triiodothyronine
NK	natural killer	**TA**	tubular atrophy
NODAT	new onset diabetes after transplant	**TACE**	trans-arterial chemo-embolisation
NSAID	non-steroidal anti-inflammatory drug	**TCR**	T cell receptor
ODR	organ donor register	**TGF**	transforming growth factor
PA	pulmonary artery	**TIA**	transient ischaemic attack
PAK	pancreas after kidney	**TIN**	tubulointerstitial nephritis
PAMP	pathogen-associated molecular pattern	**TLR**	toll-like receptor
PCR	polymerase chain reaction; protein–creatinine ratio	**TMR**	T cell-mediated rejection
PD	peritoneal dialysis	**TNF**	tumour necrosis factor
PN	parenteral nutrition	**TPG**	transpulmonary pressure gradient
PRA	panel reactive antibodies	**TPMT**	thiopurine S-methyltransferase
PTA	pancreas transplant alone	**TPR**	total peripheral resistance
PTC	peritubular capillary	**US**	ultrasound
PTH	parathyroid hormone	**VAD**	ventricular assist device
PTLD	post-transplant lymphoproliferative disease	**VRE**	vancomycin-resistant enterococci
PVD	peripheral vascular disease	**VZV**	varicella zoster virus
PVR	pulmonary vascular resistance		

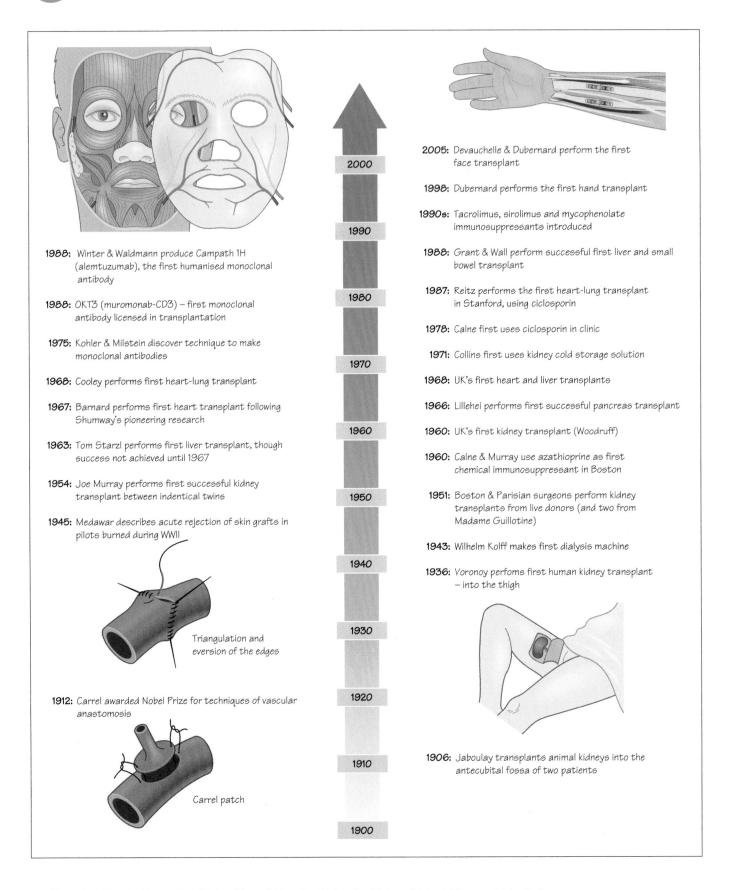

1988: Winter & Waldmann produce Campath 1H (alemtuzumab), the first humanised monoclonal antibody

1988: OKT3 (muromonab-CD3) – first monoclonal antibody licensed in transplantation

1975: Kohler & Milstein discover technique to make monoclonal antibodies

1968: Cooley performs first heart-lung transplant

1967: Barnard performs first heart transplant following Shumway's pioneering research

1963: Tom Starzl performs first liver transplant, though success not achieved until 1967

1954: Joe Murray performs first successful kidney transplant between indentical twins

1945: Medawar describes acute rejection of skin grafts in pilots burned during WWII

Triangulation and eversion of the edges

1912: Carrel awarded Nobel Prize for techniques of vascular anastomosis

Carrel patch

2000

1990

1980

1970

1960

1950

1940

1930

1920

1910

1900

2005: Devauchelle & Dubernard perform the first face transplant

1998: Dubernard performs the first hand transplant

1990s: Tacrolimus, sirolimus and mycophenolate immunosuppressants introduced

1988: Grant & Wall perform successful first liver and small bowel transplant

1987: Reitz performs the first heart-lung transplant in Stanford, using ciclosporin

1978: Calne first uses ciclosporin in clinic

1971: Collins first uses kidney cold storage solution

1968: UK's first heart and liver transplants

1966: Lillehei performs first successful pancreas transplant

1960: UK's first kidney transplant (Woodruff)

1960: Calne & Murray use azathioprine as first chemical immunosuppressant in Boston

1951: Boston & Parisian surgeons perform kidney transplants from live donors (and two from Madame Guillotine)

1943: Wilhelm Kolff makes first dialysis machine

1936: Voronoy perfoms first human kidney transplant – into the thigh

1906: Jaboulay transplants animal kidneys into the antecubital fossa of two patients

Transplantation at a Glance, First Edition. Menna Clatworthy, Christopher Watson, Michael Allison and John Dark.
10

Fundamentals

Vascular anastomoses

Transplantation of any organ demands the ability to join blood vessels together without clot formation. Early attempts inverted the edges of the vessels, as is done in bowel surgery, and thrombosis was common. It wasn't until the work of Jaboulay and Carrel that eversion of the edges was shown to overcome the early thrombotic problems, work that earned Alexis Carrel the Nobel Prize in 1912. Carrel also described two other techniques that are employed today, namely triangulation to avoid narrowing an anastomosis and the use of a patch of neighbouring vessel wall as a flange to facilitate sewing, now known as a Carrel patch.

Source of organs

Having established how to perform the operation, the next step to advance transplantation was to find suitable organs. It was in the field of renal transplantation that progress was made, albeit slowly. In Vienna in 1902, Ulrich performed an experimental kidney transplant between dogs, and four years later in 1906, Jaboulay anastomosed animal kidneys to the brachial artery in the antecubital fossa of two patients with renal failure.

Clinical transplantation was attempted during the first half of the 20th century, but was restricted by an ignorance of the importance of minimising ischaemia – some of the early attempts used kidneys from cadavers several hours, and occasionally days, after death. It wasn't until the mid-1950s that surgeons used 'fresh' organs, either from live patients who were having kidneys removed for transplantation or other reasons, or in Paris, from recently guillotined prisoners.

Where to place the kidney

Voronoy, a Russian surgeon in Kiev, is credited with the first human-to-human kidney transplant in 1936. He transplanted patients who had renal failure due to ingestion of mercuric chloride; the transplants never worked, in part because of the lengthy warm ischaemia of the kidneys (hours). Voronoy transplanted kidneys into the thigh, attracted by the easy exposure of the femoral vessels to which the renal vessels could be anastomosed. Hume, working in Boston in the early 1950s, also transplanted kidneys into the thigh, with the ureter opening on to the skin to allow ready observation of renal function. It was René Küss in Paris who, in 1951, placed the kidney intra-abdominally into the iliac fossa and established the technique used today for transplanting the kidney.

Early transplants

The 1950s was the decade that saw kidney transplantation become a reality. The alternative, dialysis, was still in its infancy so the reward for a successful transplant was enormous. Pioneers in the US and Europe, principally in Boston and Paris, vied to perform the first long-term successful transplant, but although initial function was now being achieved with 'fresh' kidneys, they rarely lasted more than a few weeks. Carrel in 1914 recognised that the immune system, the 'reaction of an organism against the foreign tissue', was the only hurdle left to be surmounted. The breakthrough in clinical transplantation came in December 1954, when a team in Boston led by Joseph Murray performed a transplant between identical twins, so bypassing the immune system completely and

demonstrating that long-term survival was possible. The kidney recipient, Richard Herrick, survived 8 years following the transplant, dying from recurrent disease; his twin brother Ronald died in 2011, 56 years later. This success was followed by more identical-twin transplants, with Woodruff performing the first in the UK in Edinburgh in 1960.

Development of immunosuppression

Demonstration that good outcomes following kidney transplantation were achievable led to exploration of ways to enable transplants between non-identical individuals. Early efforts focused on total body irradiation, but the side effects were severe and long-term results poor. The anticancer drug 6-mercaptopurine (6-MP) was shown by Calne to be immunosuppressive in dogs, but its toxicity led to the evaluation of its derivative, azathioprine. Azathioprine was used in clinical kidney transplantation in 1960 and, in combination with prednisolone, became the mainstay of immunosuppression until the 1980s, when ciclosporin was introduced. It was Roy Calne who was also responsible for the introduction of ciclosporin into clinical transplantation, the drug having originally been developed as an antifungal drug, but shelved by Sandoz, the pharmaceutical company involved, as ineffective. Jean Borel, working for Sandoz, had shown it to permit skin transplantation between mice, but Sandoz could foresee no use for such an agent. Calne confirmed the immunosuppressive properties of the drug in rodents, dogs and then humans. With ciclosporin, clinical transplantation was transformed. For the first time a powerful immunosuppressant with limited toxicity was available, and a drug that permitted successful non-renal transplantation.

Non-renal organ transplants

Transplantation of non-renal organs is an order of magnitude more difficult than transplantation of the kidney; for liver, heart or lungs the patient's own organs must first be removed before the new organs are transplanted; in kidney transplantation the native kidneys are usually left in situ.

After much pioneering experimental work by Norman Shumway to establish the operative technique, it was Christiaan Barnard who performed the first heart transplant in 1967 in South Africa. The following year the first heart was transplanted in the UK by Donald Ross, also a South African; and 1968 also saw Denton Cooley perform the first heart-lung transplant.

The first human liver transplantation was performed by Tom Starzl in Denver in 1963, the culmination of much experimental work. Roy Calne performed the first liver transplant in the UK, something that was lost in the press at the time, since Ross's heart transplant was carried out on the same day.

Although short-term survival (days) was shown to be possible, it was not until the advent of ciclosporin that clinical heart, lung and liver transplantation became a realistic therapeutic option. The immunosuppressive requirements of intestinal transplants are an order of magnitude greater, and their success had to await the advent of tacrolimus.

In addition, it should be remembered that at the time the pioneers were operating there were no brainstem criteria for the diagnosis of death, and the circulation had stopped some time before the organs were removed for transplantation.

2 Diagnosis of death and its physiology

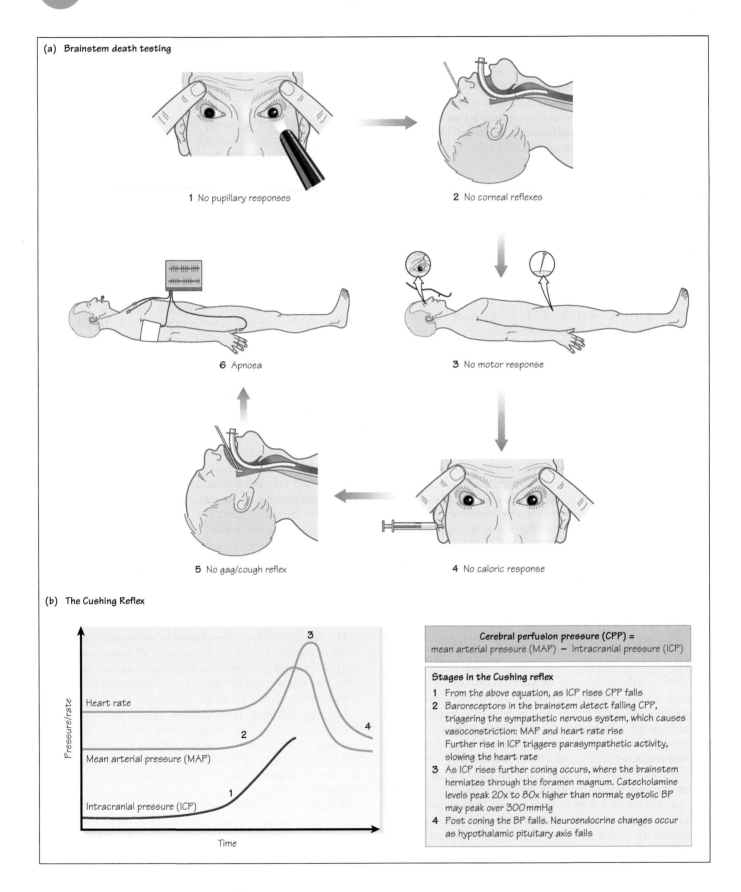

(a) Brainstem death testing

1 No pupillary responses

2 No corneal reflexes

6 Apnoea

3 No motor response

5 No gag/cough reflex

4 No caloric response

(b) The Cushing Reflex

Heart rate

Mean arterial pressure (MAP)

Intracranial pressure (ICP)

Pressure/rate

Time

Cerebral perfusion pressure (CPP) =
mean arterial pressure (MAP) − Intracranial pressure (ICP)

Stages in the Cushing reflex

1 From the above equation, as ICP rises CPP falls
2 Baroreceptors in the brainstem detect falling CPP, triggering the sympathetic nervous system, which causes vasoconstriction: MAP and heart rate rise
   Further rise in ICP triggers parasympathetic activity, slowing the heart rate
3 As ICP rises further coning occurs, where the brainstem herniates through the foramen magnum. Catecholamine levels peak 20x to 80x higher than normal; systolic BP may peak over 300 mmHg
4 Post coning the BP falls. Neuroendocrine changes occur as hypothalamic pituitary axis fails

Transplantation at a Glance, First Edition. Menna Clatworthy, Christopher Watson, Michael Allison and John Dark.

Diagnosing death

Circulatory death

Traditionally, death has been certified by the absence of a circulation, usually taken as the point at which the heart stops beating. In the UK, current guidance suggests that death may be confirmed after 5 minutes of observation following cessation of cardiac function (e.g. absence of heart sounds, absence of palpable central pulse or asystole on a continuous electrocardiogram). Organ donation after circulatory death (DCD) may occur following confirmation that death has occurred (also called non-heart-beating donation).

There are two sorts of DCD donation, controlled and uncontrolled.

Controlled DCD donation occurs when life-sustaining treatment is withdrawn on an intensive therapy unit (ITU). This usually involves discontinuing inotropes and other medicines, and stopping ventilation. This is done with the transplant team ready in the operating theatre able to proceed with organ retrieval as soon as death is confirmed.

Uncontrolled DCD donation occurs when a patient is brought into hospital and, in spite of attempts at resuscitation, dies. Since such events are unpredictable a surgical team is seldom present or prepared, and longer periods of warm ischaemia occur (see later).

Brainstem death

Brainstem death (often termed simply brain death) evolved not for the purposes of transplantation, but following technological advances in the 1960s and 1970s that enabled patients to be supported for long periods on a ventilator while deep in coma. There was a requirement to diagnose death in such patients whose cardiorespiratory function was supported artificially. Before brainstem death can be diagnosed, five pre-requisites must be met.

Pre-requisites before brainstem death testing can occur

1 The patient's condition should be due to irreversible brain damage of known aetiology.
2 There should be no evidence that the comatose state is due to depressant drugs – drug levels should be measured if doubt exists.
3 Hypothermia as a cause of coma has been excluded – the temperature should be >34°C before testing.
4 Potentially reversible circulatory, metabolic and endocrine causes have been excluded. The commonest confounding problem is hypernatraemia, which develops as a consequence of diabetes insipidus, itself induced by failure of hypothalamic antidiuretic hormone (ADH) production.
5 Potentially reversible causes of apnoea have been excluded, such as neuromuscular blocking drugs or cervical cord injury.

Tests of brainstem function

1 Pupils are fixed and unresponsive to sharp changes in the intensity of incident light.
2 The corneal reflex is absent.
3 There is no motor response within the cranial nerve distribution to adequate stimulation of any somatic area, such as elicited by supra-orbital pressure.
4 The oculo-vestibular reflexes are absent: at least 50 ml of ice-cold water is injected into each external auditory meatus. In life, the gaze moves to the side of injection; in death, there is no movement.
5 There is no cough reflex to bronchial stimulation, e.g. to a suction catheter passed down the trachea to the carina, or gag response to stimulation of the posterior pharynx with a spatula.
6 The apnoea test: following pre-oxygenation with 100% oxygen, the respiratory rate is lowered until the pCO_2 rises above $6.0\,kPa$ (with a pH less than 7.4). The patient is then disconnected from the ventilator and observed for 5 minutes for a respiratory response. Following brainstem death spinal reflexes may still be intact, resulting in movements of the limbs and torso.

These criteria are used in the UK; different criteria exist elsewhere in the world, some countries requiring an unresponsive electroencephalogram (EEG) or demonstration of no flow in the cerebral arteries on angiography. The UK criteria assess brainstem function without which independent life is not possible.

Causes of death

Most organ donors have died from an intracranial catastrophe of some sort, be it haemorrhage, thrombosis, hypoxia, trauma or tumour. The past decade has seen a change in the types of brain injury suffered by deceased organ donors; deaths due to trauma are much less common, and have been replaced by an increased prevalence of deaths from stroke. This is also a reflection of the increased age of organ donors today.

Physiology of brainstem death

Cushing's reflex and the catecholamine storm

Because the skull is a rigid container of fixed volume, the swelling that follows a brain injury results in increased intracranial pressure (ICP). The perfusion pressure of the brain is the mean arterial pressure (MAP) minus the ICP, hence as ICP rises, MAP must rise to maintain perfusion. This is triggered by baroreceptors in the brainstem that activate the autonomic nervous system, resulting in catecholamine release. Catecholamine levels may reach 20-fold those of normal, with systemic blood pressure rising dramatically.

The 'catecholamine storm' has deleterious effects on other organs: the left ventricle is placed under significant strain with subendocardial haemorrhage, and subintimal haemorrhage occur in arteries, particularly at the points of bifurcation, predisposing to thrombosis of the organ following transplantation; perfusion of the abdominal organs suffers in response to the high catecholamine levels. Eventually the swollen brain forces the brainstem to herniate down through the foramen magnum (coning), an occurrence that is marked by its compression of the oculomotor nerve and resultant pupillary dilatation. Once coning has occurred circulatory collapse follows with hypotension, secondary myocardial depression and vasodilatation, with failure of hormonal and neural regulators of vascular tone.

Decompressive craniectomy

Modern neurosurgical practices include craniectomy (removal of parts of the skull) to allow the injured brain to swell, reducing ICP and so maintaining cerebral perfusion. While such practices may protect the brainstem, the catastrophic nature of the brain injury may be such that recovery will not occur and prolongation of treatment will be inappropriate. Such is the setting in which DCD donation often takes place.

Neuroendocrine changes associated with brain death

Following brainstem death a number of neuroendocrine changes occur, most notably the cessation of ADH secretion, resulting in diabetes insipidus and consequent hypernatraemia. This is treated by the administration of exogenous ADH and 5% dextrose. Other components of the hypothalamic-pituitary axis may also merit treatment to optimise the organs, including the administration of glucocorticoids and triiodothyronine (T3).

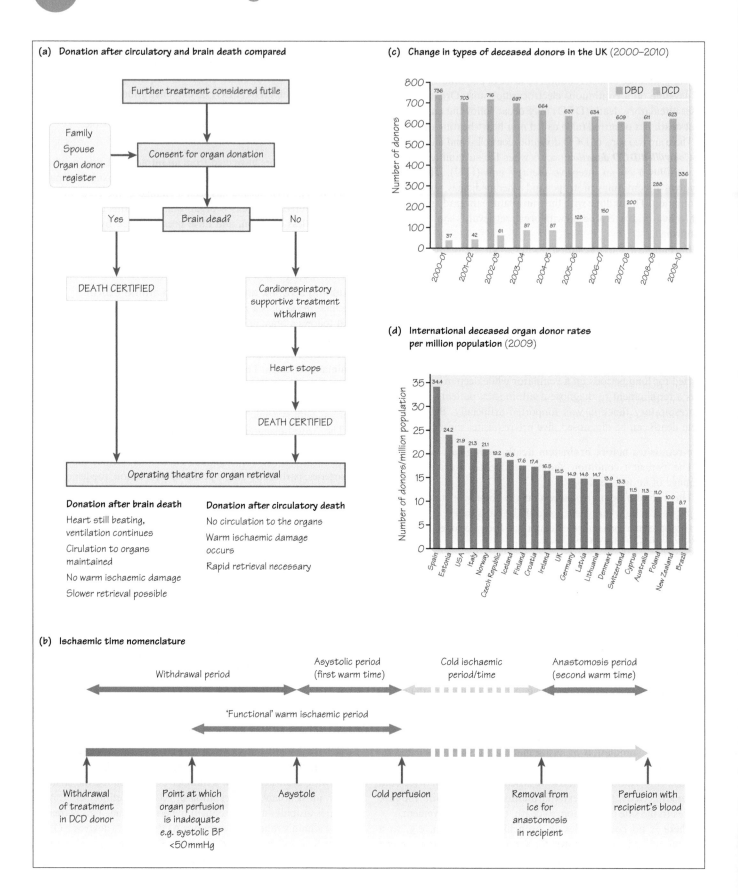

(a) Donation after circulatory and brain death compared

Further treatment considered futile

Family
Spouse
Organ donor register → Consent for organ donation

Yes ← Brain dead? → No

DEATH CERTIFIED

Cardiorespiratory supportive treatment withdrawn

Heart stops

DEATH CERTIFIED

Operating theatre for organ retrieval

Donation after brain death

Heart still beating, ventilation continues

Cirulation to organs maintained

No warm ischaemic damage

Slower retrieval possible

Donation after circulatory death

No circulation to the organs

Warm ischaemic damage occurs

Rapid retrieval necessary

(c) Change in types of deceased donors in the UK (2000–2010)

■ DBD ■ DCD

(d) International deceased organ donor rates per million population (2009)

(b) Ischaemic time nomenclature

Withdrawal period

Asystolic period (first warm time)

Cold ischaemic period/time

Anastomosis period (second warm time)

'Functional' warm ischaemic period

Withdrawal of treatment in DCD donor

Point at which organ perfusion is inadequate e.g. systolic BP <50mmHg

Asystole

Cold perfusion

Removal from ice for anastomosis in recipient

Perfusion with recipient's blood

Transplantation at a Glance, First Edition. Menna Clatworthy, Christopher Watson, Michael Allison and John Dark.

Opting in or opting out?

In the UK, as in most countries in the world, the next of kin are approached for consent/authorisation for organ donation, a system known colloquially as 'opting in'. This system is facilitated by having a register, such as the UK organ donor register (ODR), where people can register their wishes to be a donor when they die; 29% of the UK population are on the register. However, opinion polls show that nearer to 90% of people are in favour of organ donation, suggesting that the shortfall is a consequence of apathy. When a person is on the ODR the relatives are much more likely (>90%) to consent to donation than where the wishes of the deceased were not known (~60%).

In some parts of the world, most notably Spain, a system of presumed consent exists where you are presumed to have wanted to be an organ donor unless you registered your wish in life not to be so, i.e. you 'opted out'. Spain also has the highest donation rate in the world, so on the face of it a switch to opting in should improve donation. However, there are other points to consider.
- Spain had presumed consent for 10 years before its donation rate rose – only after reorganising the transplant coordination infrastructure did donation rates rise, and it has been argued that it was this, not presumed consent, that was the key factor.
- Even in Spain, the relatives are asked for permission and their wishes observed.
- Other reasons that Spain has a higher donation rate than the UK include using organs from a wider age range, with many more donors over 60 and 70 being used than in the UK.
- Some countries with presumed consent, such as Sweden, have donation rates below that of the UK.

Patterns of organ donation

The past decade has seen an increase in the number of deceased organ donors in the UK. That increase has been due to a 10-fold increase in DCD donors, who now comprise a third of all deceased donors in the UK. The number of donation after brain death (DBD) donors has fallen, although the proportion of potential DBD donors for whom consent for donation is obtained has increased.

Organ retrieval

DBD donation

Since DBD donors are certified dead while on cardiorespiratory support, the organs continue to be perfused with oxygenated blood while the retrieval surgery takes place. Once the dissection phase is completed, ice-cold preservation solution is passed through a cannula into the aorta with exsanguination via the vena cava; at the same time ice-cold cardioplegia is perfused into the coronary arteries to arrest the heart. The organs are flushed and cooled in situ, removed and then placed into more preservation solution and packaged for transit in crushed ice.

DCD donation

In contrast to DBD donation, the circulation has, by definition, already ceased in DCD donors before organ retrieval commences. In controlled DCD donation, the surgical team is ready and waiting in the theatre, while treatment is withdrawn either in the ITU or in the theatre complex. Death may then be instantaneous, but more commonly follows a variable period of time while the blood pressure falls before cardiac arrest occurs. When the blood pressure is insufficient to perfuse the vital organs, functional warm ischaemia commences. In the UK no treatment can be given to the donor prior to death; in the US it is permissible to give heparin to prevent in situ thrombosis. When the retrieval surgery begins the organs are still warm and already ischaemic. Unlike DBD donation, where the organs are mobilised while a circulation is still present, for DCD donation the abdominal organs are perfused with cold preservation solution as soon as the abdomen is opened, to convert warm ischaemia to cold ischaemia; once cooled the organs are rapidly mobilised and removed.

Ischaemic times

The nomenclature used for the time periods from donation to transplantation is shown in Figure 3c. Warm ischaemia is most deleterious to an organ, and it is often said that a minute of warm ischaemia does the same damage as an hour of cold ischaemia. Since the duration of ischaemia is one of the few things that a surgeon can modify to improve the outcome following transplantation, every effort is made to minimise both warm and cold ischaemia and to transplant the organs as soon as possible.

Contraindications to donation

It has long been established that malignancy and infection can be transferred with a donor organ to the recipient. However, there are occasions, such as when a potential recipient will die if not transplanted immediately, where the balance of risks may favour using at-risk organs. Nevertheless the following are generally considered contraindications to donation:
- active cancer, except skin cancer (not melanoma) and some primary brain tumours; this includes recently treated cancers;
- untreated systemic infection;
- hepatitis B or C or HIV, except to similarly infected recipients;
- other rare viral infections, e.g. rabies.

At the time of retrieval the donor surgeon must do a thorough laparotomy and thoracotomy looking for evidence of occult malignancy, such as a lung, stomach, oesophageal or pancreatic tumour. In addition, it goes without saying that evidence of severe, permanent damage to the organ to be transplanted is a contraindication to its use, e.g. a heart with coronary artery disease or a cirrhotic liver.

Suboptimal organs

Less than ideal organs, sometimes called expanded criteria or marginal organs, are those whose anticipated function is likely to be less than ideal, but nevertheless adequate. Every recipient would like a new organ, but the reality is that all organs are 'second hand', and someone dying below the age of 60 usually has significant other comorbidity that contributed to their early death, such as cigarette smoking-associated pathologies or hypertension. Deaths from trauma are increasingly uncommon. The severe shortage of organs, particularly from young donors, means that compromises have to be made to balance the risks of dying on the waiting list: 25% of patients awaiting a lung transplant will die in the first year of waiting, as will 15% of those awaiting a liver.

4 Live donor kidney transplantation

Types of living donors

1 Related

Most commonly parent to child or sibling to sibling

2 Unrelated

Usually spouse to spouse, most commonly wife to husband. Occasionally close friends donate kidneys

3 Altruistic

Recently introduced in the UK (2007). Members of the general public may give a kidney to someone on the waiting list. The same work-up applies as with any other living donor, with particular emphasis on lack of psychiatric condition and on ensuring the individual is fully aware of the implications of their action

Assessment of living donors

Donor–recipient compatibility
- ABO
- HLA

Donor psychosocial wellbeing

Past medical history
- Previous renal disease
- Diseases associated with CKD, e.g. DM or hypertension
- Bladder/prostate problems

Investigations
- Urine dipstick
- Quantification of proteinuria
- GFR/creatinine clearance
- Split kidney function
- Renal anatomy (US/MRI scan)

Donor medical fitness
- Respiratory (CXR)
- Cardiovascular (ECG, ECHO, stress test)
- Infections (Hep B/C, HIV)
- Body mass index

Exclusion criteria for living donors

1. Psycho-social factors
- Inadequately treated psychiatric condition
- Active drug or alcohol abuse
- Inadequate cognitive capacity

2. Renal disease
- Evidence of renal disease (low GFR, proteinuria, haematuria, known GN)
- Recurrent nephrolithiasis or bilateral kidney stones
- Significant abnormal renal anatomy

3. Other medical problems
- Diabetes mellitus
- Hyertension (relative contraindication)
- Collagen vascular disease
- Prior MI or treated coronary artery disease
- Significant pulmonary disease
- Current or previous malignancy
- Significant hepatic disease
- Significant neurological disease
- Morbid obesity

4. Infection
- Active infection
- Chronic viral infection (HIV, Hep B/C)

Transplantation at a Glance, First Edition. Menna Clatworthy, Christopher Watson, Michael Allison and John Dark.

The limited supply of deceased donor organs and an ever-increasing number of patients waiting for kidney transplantation has led to the widespread use of living donors. Renal transplantation has the unique advantage, compared with other organs, that most individuals have two kidneys, and if not diseased, have sufficient reserve of renal function to survive unimpeded with a single kidney. The shortage of donors has also led to the use of parts of non-paired organs, such as liver and lung lobes, the tail of pancreas and lengths of intestine from living donors; indeed, even live donation of the heart has occurred, when the donor has lung disease and received a combined heart-lung transplant, with their own heart being transplanted to someone else, so called 'domino transplantation'. For the purposes of this chapter we will focus on live kidney donation, but similar principles apply to other organs.

Advantages of living donor transplantation

1 Living donation is an elective operation that takes place during standard working hours, when there is a full complement of staff and back-up facilities immediately available, minimising peri-operative complications. This is in contrast to deceased donor transplants, which often occur at night as an emergency procedure.
2 The donor kidney function and anatomy can be fully assessed prior to transplantation. This ensures that the kidney, once transplanted, will provide the recipient with an adequate glomerular filtration rate (GFR) post-transplant.
3 The donor nephrectomy and recipient transplant operation can take place in adjacent theatres to minimise the cold ischaemic time.
4 Unlike deceased donor organs, there has been no agonal phase, no catecholamine storm and no other peri-mortem injury to affect the function of the kidney.
5 Allograft survival. Unsurprisingly, given the considerations listed in 1–4, allograft survival is better in living donor kidneys compared with deceased donor kidneys. For example, in the UK, the 5-year survival of a living donor kidney is around 89% compared with 82% for a deceased donor kidney (1999–2003 cohort).

Living kidney donation

Assessing a living kidney donor

Medical fitness of donor

Donating a kidney involves a significant operation, lasting 1 to 3 hours. A detailed history and careful examination should be performed. If the donor has any pre-existing medical condition that would place them at high risk of complications during an anaesthetic, e.g. previous myocardial infarction (MI) or poor left ventricular (LV) function, then they would not be suitable for donation. A full examination is performed, including assessment of the donor's body mass index (BMI). Typical donor investigations would include a full blood count, clotting screen, renal function tests, liver function tests, an ECG and a chest radiograph; a more detailed cardiological work-up including echocardiogram and cardiac stress testing are performed if indicated. Tests to exclude chronic viral infections such as hepatitis B and C, and HIV are also performed.

Psychosocial fitness

As well as physical considerations, the transplant clinicians must also be sure that the donor is mentally and emotionally sound and understands the implications of the procedure. They must be certain that there is no coercion involved. Donors are also assessed by an independent third party.

Adequacy of donor renal function

Donation will involve the donor losing one kidney. Thus it is important to ensure that the donor has sufficient renal reserve to allow this to occur and leave adequate renal function for a healthy existence.

History: Pre-existing medical conditions, such as diabetes mellitus or hypertension, which can lead to chronic kidney disease are a relative contraindication to donation. A family history of renal disease should also be sought, e.g. polycystic kidney disease, Alport's syndrome or a familial glomerulonephritis.

Examination: Hypertension may be previously undiagnosed and should therefore be carefully assessed on more than one occasion.

Investigations: Initially, an ultrasound scan of the renal tract is performed to ensure that the donor has two kidneys of normal size. The urine is tested to ensure no microscopic haematuria or proteinuria, which may indicate underlying renal disease. Quantification of urinary protein with a spot urine protein–creatinine ratio, an albumin–creatinine ratio or a 24-hour urine collection for protein is also required. Renal function is estimated by serum creatinine, creatinine clearance and measured GFR, together with the split function. If the renal function is sufficient to allow halving of the GFR and some decline in renal function with age, then the donor is considered suitable. Renal anatomy is defined by magnetic resonance (MR) or computed tomography (CT) scan to allow choice of the most suitable kidney to remove – preference is for the kidney with single artery and vein; if otherwise equal, the left kidney is removed since it has a longer vein to facilitate implantation.

Compatibility

• **ABO:** The blood group of the donor must be compatible with the recipient. Transplantation of an incompatible blood group kidney can lead to hyperacute rejection if an individual has preformed antibodies. ABO incompatible transplantation is possible, but the recipient must have the antibodies removed either by antigen-specific columns or by plasma exchange; enhanced immunosuppression is usually required.
• **HLA:** HLA matching is associated with prolonged graft survival, but even the worst-matched live donor kidney is superior to the best-matched deceased donor kidney. Where several donors come forward the best match is chosen. If the prospective recipient has antibodies to HLA antigens on the donor, the recipient may undergo antibody removal therapy. However, it tends to be more difficult to remove HLA antibodies and results of HLA-incompatible transplantation are inferior to those of ABO incompatible transplantation.

Donor nephrectomy technique

Donor nephrectomy was traditionally an open procedure, but is now done laparoscopically in most centres. An open nephrectomy is performed either through modified flank incision or a subcostal incision. Careful dissection is required to preserve the main vessels and ureteric blood supply. The advantage of an open approach is that it minimises potential abdominal complications intra-operatively. However, it leaves a significant surgical scar (which can develop herniation in the longer term) and requires a longer period of recovery (6–8 weeks). In contrast, a laparoscopic approach is technically more demanding, may take longer to perform, but leaves a smaller surgical scar. The average inpatient stay is just 2–4 days, and recovery time much shorter.

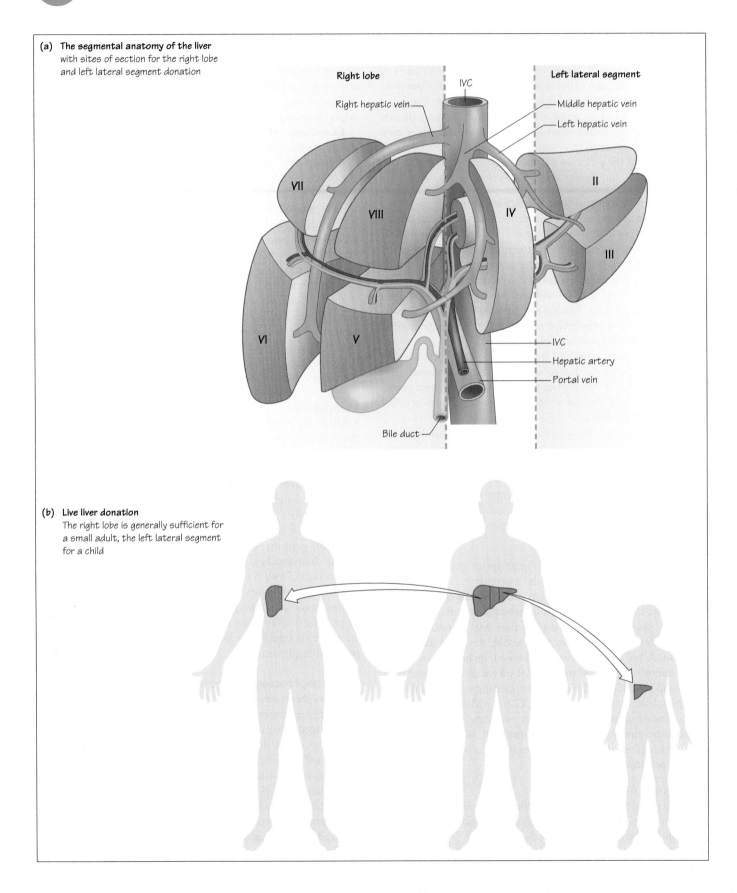

(a) The segmental anatomy of the liver
with sites of section for the right lobe
and left lateral segment donation

Right lobe

IVC

Right hepatic vein

Left lateral segment

Middle hepatic vein

Left hepatic vein

VII

VIII

IV

II

III

VI

V

IVC

Hepatic artery

Portal vein

Bile duct

(b) Live liver donation
The right lobe is generally sufficient for
a small adult, the left lateral segment
for a child

Transplantation at a Glance, First Edition. Menna Clatworthy, Christopher Watson, Michael Allison and John Dark.

Live liver donation

Much of what has been said about the assessment of a kidney donor applies to a liver donor, with the exception that the full assessment of the liver, its function, exclusion of disease and assessment of its anatomy are paramount.

The clinical imperative to donate

Unlike kidney transplantation, where the alternative of dialysis will keep a potential recipient alive, there is no fall back to liver transplantation. If a patient is deemed to require a liver transplant then they have a 10–20% chance of dying while waiting for a deceased donor; if they require an urgent liver transplant the chance of death is higher. It is against this background that potential donors are approached, in the knowledge that the clinical situation is often coercive by its very nature. There is not the luxury of time to assess the potential donor, unlike with live kidney donation.

In addition, a further imperative may be added. For some conditions, such as large primary liver tumours, liver transplantation is not considered to be a sensible use of deceased donor organs because the chance of 5-year survival is less than 50%. It has been proposed that live donors should be allowed to donate in such circumstances, although there is an ethical distinction between putting your life at risk to donate a liver lobe in the expectation of a good outcome compared with an expectation that life may only be prolonged for a year or so.

Live donor liver surgery

Principles

Following resection of a part of the liver, the remaining liver will grow relatively quickly to fill the space previously occupied by the resected portion. The process of dividing the liver into two is difficult, since there are no clear anatomical planes to follow. The blood supply and bile ducts come into the hilum and divide, giving branches to each of the eight segments; the blood drains through the hepatic veins, which, in part, run at right-angles to the inflow vessels.

Two separate resections may be performed.

Left lateral segment

The left lateral segment of the liver (segments 2 and 3) can be removed relatively easily, leaving a single portal vein, hepatic artery, hepatic vein and bile duct on the donated liver. The volume of the left lobe makes it suitable only for use in a child.

Full right lobe

The right lobe of the liver comprises segments 5 to 8. It is marked on the surface of the liver by a line from the gall bladder fundus to the suprahepatic inferior vena cava (IVC), a line of division that runs almost on top of the middle hepatic vein. By dividing the liver along this plane the arterial inflow and biliary drainage are separated. However, the middle hepatic vein, which drains segment 4 as well as segments 5 and 8, needs to be taken either with the donated liver or left in the recipient, with venous drainage from the other half being reconstructed using donor saphenous vein to prevent infarction of the segment.

In both cases the liver is removed from the IVC, leaving that with the donor and necessitating that the recipient undergoes a hepatectomy with caval conservation.

Recipient suitability

Not all recipients will be suitable for a live donor transplant, either because they are too big, or for anatomical or pathological reasons.

Live liver donor assessment

Assessment of the potential donor

Liver resection is a much bigger procedure than nephrectomy and demands a greater level of fitness. Careful history taking and clinical examination are paramount, particularly with respect to exercise tolerance.

- *Cardiac screening:* echo, stress test (echo or nuclear medicine).
- *Respiratory:* chest radiograph; pulmonary function tests if concern exists.
- *Psychiatric:* careful assessment, particularly because of the issues mentioned earlier with respect to coercion, albeit through a sense of obligation.

Assessment of liver function

Standard screening tests for underlying liver disease are performed on the potential donor, similar to those that form the assessment of any patient presenting with newly diagnosed liver disease. An ultrasound of liver and spleen is performed to screen for patency of the vessels and evidence of portal hypertension. Any intrahepatic lesion is appropriately characterised. Biopsy may be required to fully evaluate the liver.

The most important aspect of live donation is to estimate the volume of the liver that can be safely donated, and whether this would suffice in the recipient, leaving sufficient in the donor. In general, leaving less than 30% of viable donor liver behind is unsafe, and more is required if part of the residual liver will be rendered ischaemic by the procedure, such as when the middle hepatic vein drainage of segment 4 is lost. The recipient requires a graft estimated to be >0.8% of their body weight.

Assessment of liver anatomy

The anatomy of the liver varies. Normally the arterial supply to the right lobe of the liver comes from the right branch of the hepatic artery, and that to the left comes from the left branch; unfortunately this is not always the case, with segmental vessels to the right lobe sometimes arising from the left hepatic artery, and vice versa. An accessory left hepatic artery arising from the left gastric artery or an accessory or replaced right hepatic artery arising from the superior mesenteric artery may be present. Segmental bile ducts may be similarly errant in their obedience of anatomical principles. Careful elucidation of anatomy usually requires MR imaging together with intraoperative ultrasound prior to resection. Significant abnormalities may preclude donation.

Risks of donation

Living kidney donation is an elective procedure, and the operation is associated with a low mortality rate (around 0.03%). The re-operation rate is less than 1%, and serious post-operative complications such as pulmonary embolism are uncommon (less than 3%). The long-term outcome for living donors appears to be satisfactory.

Donation of a liver lobe is more dangerous. Donation of the left lateral segment for a child has a relatively low mortality rate (0.2%) in contrast to donation of the right lobe for an adult, where the risk of death is 0.5–1%. Death is commonly related to surgical complications (bleeding), post-operative complications (pulmonary embolism) or lack of sufficient residual liver – in the latter case donors have occasionally required emergency transplantation themselves. Morbidity is around 35%, with bleeding and bile leaks (from the cut surface) common.

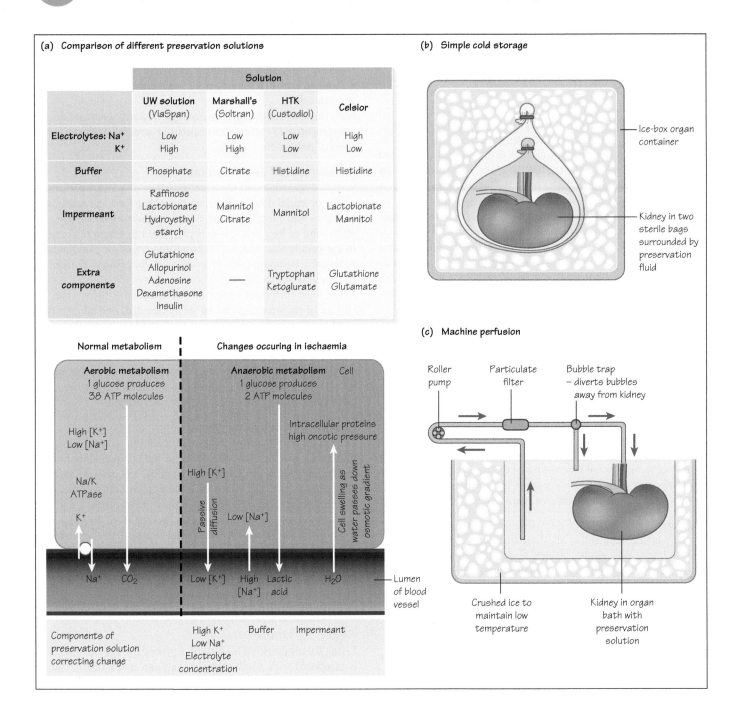

(a) Comparison of different preservation solutions

	Solution			
	UW solution (ViaSpan)	**Marshall's** (Soltran)	**HTK** (Custodiol)	**Celsior**
Electrolytes: Na⁺ **K⁺**	Low High	Low High	Low Low	High Low
Buffer	Phosphate	Citrate	Histidine	Histidine
Impermeant	Raffinose Lactobionate Hydroyethyl starch	Mannitol Citrate	Mannitol	Lactobionate Mannitol
Extra components	Glutathione Allopurinol Adenosine Dexamethasone Insulin	—	Tryptophan Ketoglurate	Glutathione Glutamate

(b) Simple cold storage

Ice-box organ container

Kidney in two sterile bags surrounded by preservation fluid

Normal metabolism | **Changes occuring in ischaemia**

Aerobic metabolism
1 glucose produces 38 ATP molecules

High [K⁺]
Low [Na⁺]

Na/K ATPase

K⁺

Na⁺ CO_2

Anaerobic metabolism   Cell
1 glucose produces 2 ATP molecules

Intracellular proteins high oncotic pressure

High [K⁺]

Passive diffusion

Low [Na⁺]

Cell swelling as water passes down osmotic gradient

Low [K⁺]   High [Na⁺]   Lactic acid H_2O — Lumen of blood vessel

| Components of preservation solution correcting change | High K⁺ Low Na⁺ Electrolyte concentration | Buffer | Impermeant |

(c) Machine perfusion

Roller pump   Particulate filter   Bubble trap – diverts bubbles away from kidney

Crushed ice to maintain low temperature   Kidney in organ bath with preservation solution

The effects of ischaemia

Cellular integrity depends on the function of membrane pumps, which maintain the intracellular ion composition. These pumps use high-energy phosphate molecules such as adenosine triphosphate (ATP) as their energy source. ATP is generated from ADP via a series of chemical reactions, which require sugars, amino acids or fatty acids as substrate. Aerobic metabolism is 19 times more efficient than anaerobic metabolism in generating ATP. ATP and other high-energy phosphate molecules are also important for other metabolic processes within a cell.

When the circulation to an organ stops, it switches from aerobic to anaerobic metabolism. Since there is no substrate reaching the cells from which ATP can be generated, cellular ATP stores rapidly deplete, membrane pumps fail and cellular integrity is lost. Other energy-dependent metabolic pathways also fail.

Transplantation at a Glance, First Edition. Menna Clatworthy, Christopher Watson, Michael Allison and John Dark.

Principles of organ preservation

Organ preservation aims to reduce the effects of ischaemic injury by a combination of cooling and use of special preservation solutions.

Cooling

Cooling an organ by 10°C halves the metabolic rate, and cooling to 4°C reduces metabolism to less than a tenth of the rate at normal body temperature. There are two ways to cool an organ, core-cooling and topical cooling. Core cooling involves flushing the organ with ice-cold preservation solution via its arterial supply. It is rapid and effective, but a large volume of fluid is needed to cool an organ quickly, since heat transfer is slow. Topical cooling involves immersing an organ in saline ice slush, or placing slush topically over the organ in the deceased donor while organ removal proceeds. Topical cooling is very inefficient compared with core cooling, and it really only works well in small children or for small organs with large surface area to volume ratio, such as the pancreas. In reality, a combination of core cooling and topical cooling are employed.

Preservation solutions

Organ preservation solutions aim to minimise the cellular changes occurring during cold storage. They comprise three principal components.

Electrolytes

The intracellular electrolyte composition is characterised by high potassium and low sodium concentrations, in contrast to the low potassium, high sodium milieu that surrounds the cells. Early preservation solutions used an electrolyte composition more akin to intracellular fluid to minimise the diffusion that occurs in the cold when the Na/K ATPase pumps fail. In fact, there appears to be no benefit in having an intracellular composition, and indeed a high potassium concentration in the preservation fluid causes vasospasm and may cause problems on reperfusion, particularly of the liver, when the preservation fluid is washed out of the organ into the circulation (it may induce ventricular arrhythmias).

Impermeants

Impermeants are osmotically active substances such as lactobionate and raffinose, which stay outside the cells and so prevent cell swelling by countering the osmotic potential of the intracellular proteins. Some solutions, such as UW solution, also contain a colloid component (hydroxyethyl starch).

Buffer

Anaerobic metabolism results in the accumulation of metabolites, including lactic acid. To keep the extracellular milieu at a fixed pH, the preservation solutions contain a buffer. The nature of the buffer varies between the different solutions.

Additional reagents

Some solutions have additional compounds that may add substrate for metabolism, scavenge harmful metabolic products, and so on.

Preservation solutions in practice

Traditionally used solutions for abdominal organs include Ross and Marshall's hypertonic citrate solution for kidneys and Belzer's University of Wisconsin (UW) solution for liver, kidney and pancreas; more recently other solutions such as Bretschneider's histidine-tryptophan-ketoglutarate (HTK) solution and Celsior have been developed as multi-organ preservation solutions. Using these solutions it is possible to keep a liver or pancreas for 18 hours and a kidney for 36 hours, although the shorter the cold ischaemic period the better (typically less than 11 hours for liver and pancreas, and less than 18 hours for a kidney).

Preservation of the heart uses high-potassium cardioplegia solutions to stop the heart, but tolerance to cold ischaemia using these electrolyte solutions is poor and cold storage of the heart beyond 4 hours is undesirable.

Preservation of the lungs is different again, and there is no clear consensus on the best perfusion fluid, though solutions with an extracellular ion composition seem to be better than the more traditional 'intracellular' fluids. Initial ischaemic injury to the lungs can be ameliorated by insufflating them with oxygen, something that has greatest benefits in lungs donated after circulatory death.

Static storage or machine perfusion

Static cold storage

The simplest method of preservation is to flush cold preservation solution through an organ, and then store the organ in preservation solution in an ice-box. It has the advantage of low cost and simplicity.

Continuous cold perfusion

An alternative for kidneys, this involves connecting the kidney to a machine that pumps ice-cold preservation solution through the artery in a circuit, thus removing waste products and providing new energy substrates. This is probably superior to static cold storage for long preservation periods, but is more costly and offers little benefit for short durations of ischaemia.

Normothermic perfusion

There has been much recent interest in creating an artificial circulation to pump oxygenated blood through an organ to keep it functioning as normal, so avoiding ischaemia. Prototypes exist for all the thoracic and abdominal organs currently transplanted.

(a) The complement pathway

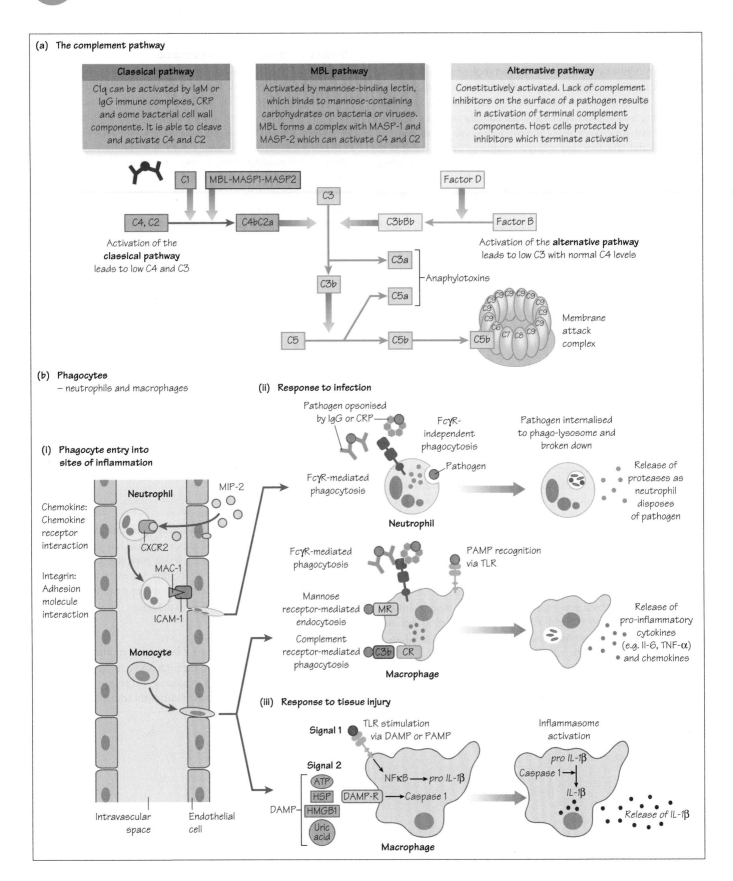

Classical pathway

C1q can be activated by IgM or IgG immune complexes, CRP and some bacterial cell wall components. It is able to cleave and activate C4 and C2

MBL pathway

Activated by mannose-binding lectin, which binds to mannose-containing carbohydrates on bacteria or viruses. MBL forms a complex with MASP-1 and MASP-2 which can activate C4 and C2

Alternative pathway

Constitutively activated. Lack of complement inhibitors on the surface of a pathogen results in activation of terminal complement components. Host cells protected by inhibitors which terminate activation

C1 · MBL-MASP1-MASP2 · C3 · Factor D

C4, C2 → C4bC2a · C3bBb ← Factor B

Activation of the **classical pathway** leads to low C4 and C3

Activation of the **alternative pathway** leads to low C3 with normal C4 levels

C3a · C5a — Anaphylotoxins

C3b

C5 → C5b → Membrane attack complex

(b) Phagocytes
— neutrophils and macrophages

(i) Phagocyte entry into sites of inflammation

Neutrophil

MIP-2

Chemokine: Chemokine receptor interaction

CXCR2

Integrin: Adhesion molecule interaction

MAC-1

ICAM-1

Monocyte

Intravascular space · Endothelial cell

(ii) Response to infection

Pathogen opsonised by IgG or CRP

FcγR-independent phagocytosis

FcγR-mediated phagocytosis

Pathogen

Pathogen internalised to phago-lysosome and broken down

Release of proteases as neutrophil disposes of pathogen

Neutrophil

FcγR-mediated phagocytosis

PAMP recognition via TLR

Mannose receptor-mediated endocytosis — MR

Complement receptor-mediated phagocytosis — C3b · CR

Macrophage

Release of pro-inflammatory cytokines (e.g. Il-6, TNF-α) and chemokines

(iii) Response to tissue injury

Signal 1 — TLR stimulation via DAMP or PAMP

Signal 2

ATP · HSP · HMGB1 · Uric acid — DAMP

DAMP-R

NFκB → pro IL-1β

→ Caspase 1

Inflammasome activation

pro IL-1β

Caspase 1 → IL-1β

Release of IL-1β

Macrophage

Transplantation at a Glance, First Edition. Menna Clatworthy, Christopher Watson, Michael Allison and John Dark.

The role of the immune system is to identify and remove invading microorganisms before they cause harm to the host. This is achieved by a rapid, non-specific innate immune response that is followed by a more finely tuned, targeted, adaptive immune response. The innate immune system is comprised of components that directly recognise and destroy pathogens (the complement system), a number of 'flags' known as opsonins (e.g. C-reactive protein [CRP], C3b, natural IgM antibody), which make pathogens more easily recognised by immune cells such as phagocytes (**neutrophils and macrophages**), which engulf and kill internalised pathogens, and natural killer (NK) cells, which can detect and destroy virus-infected cells.

The complement system

The complement system is a series of proteases, which are sequentially activated and culminate in the formation of the membrane attack complex (MAC). The MAC forms a hole in the membrane of the cell into which it is inserted (pathogen or host), disrupting membrane integrity and causing cell lysis. The complement system can be activated in three ways:

- the classical pathway
- the alternative pathway
- the mannose binding pathway.

IgM or immune complexed IgG activate the classical pathway. The alternative pathway is constitutively active, while the mannose binding pathway is activated by carbohydrates present on pathogens. The net result of activating any of the three pathways is the formation of a C3 convertase (either C4bC2a or C3bBb), which cleaves C3. The resulting C3b cleaves C5 and activates a final common pathway resulting in MAC formation. Complement activation also leads to the production of anaphylotoxins (C3a and C5a), which activate neutrophils and mast cells, promoting inflammation. In addition, C3b can opsonise pathogens for uptake by complement receptors CR1 and CR3 on phagocytes.

Pentraxins

These are a family of proteins with a pentameric structure that include CRP and serum amyloid protein (SAP). CRP and SAP are synthesised in the liver and rapidly released into the bloodstream in response to inflammation and are therefore called acute phase proteins. Pentraxins bind to phosphorylcholine found on the surface of pathogens and can fix complement (via the classical pathway) and opsonise pathogens for uptake by phagocytes through binding to surface Fc-gamma receptors (FcγRs). Pentraxins can also bind to apoptotic cells, facilitating their disposal.

Phagocytes

Phagocytes (from the Greek word 'phagein' – 'to eat') are cells that ingest debris, pathogens and dying cells. There are two main types of phagocyte, neutrophils (which circulate in the blood until they are called into tissues), and macrophages, which are resident in tissues and act as immune sentinels. The circulating monocyte is the precursor to tissue macrophages. Neutrophils are the most abundant circulating leucocyte and can be identified by their multi-lobed nucleus and the presence of numerous granules within their cytoplasm, which contain proteases (for example myeloperoxidase) and other bacteriocidal substances. Neutrophils move into tissues by virtue of surface molecules called integrins (for example MAC-1), which bind to adhesion molecules that are upregulated on vascular endothelium in inflamed tissue (for example ICAM-1).

Phagocytes detect pathogens via membrane receptors, which recognise repeating surface motifs on microbes, so-called pathogen-associated molecular patterns (PAMPs). These innate receptors include the toll-like receptors (TLRs) and the mannose receptors. Phagocytes can also internalise opsonised pathogens via complement receptors and FcγRs. Once internalised, the microbe will be destroyed within the phagolysosome by proteases and by the generation of oxygen and nitrogen free radicals. Tissue-resident macrophages secrete pro-inflammatory cytokines such as tumour necrosis factor (TNF)-α and interleukin (IL)-6, which lead to changes in vascular permeability, and in the molecules expressed on vascular endothelial cells. They also produce chemicals that attract neutrophils and monocytes (known as chemokines). These changes facilitate the entry of neutrophils and monocytes from the circulation into the site of infection and result in the cardinal signs of inflammation (calor, dolor, rubor and tumor, i.e. heat, pain, redness and swelling).

Macrophages can also be activated by danger/damage-associated molecular patterns (DAMPs), for example heat shock proteins (HSPs) or ATP, which are release by damaged or dying host cells. This leads to activation of the inflammasome and the production of IL1-β and IL18.

In addition, macrophages have the capacity to process and present antigen (see Chapter 8).

Mast cells

Mast cells are large tissue-resident cells found mainly in the skin and at mucosal surfaces. They are packed with granules containing vasoactive amines (e.g. histamine) and heparin. Mast cell degranulation may be induced by trauma or UV light, and by binding of IgE antibodies to Fc-epsilon receptors found on the surface of mast cells. Mast cells play an important role in allergy and anaphylaxis.

Natural killer cells

Natural killer cells express surface receptors (killer-cell immunoglobulin-like receptors [KIRs]), which bind to and assess cell surface major histocompatibility complex (MHC) class I molecules. If non-self or altered self-antigen is detected on class I molecules, e.g. in virally infected cells or tumour cells, then the NK cell will destroy this cell by the release of perforin (punches holes in cells), granzyme (poisons cells) or the induction of apoptosis. In addition, NK cells express FcγRs and can therefore be activated against antibody-opsonised cells. This is known as antibody-dependent cellular cytotoxicity (ADCC).

8 Adaptive immunity and antigen presentation

(a) Adaptive immunity

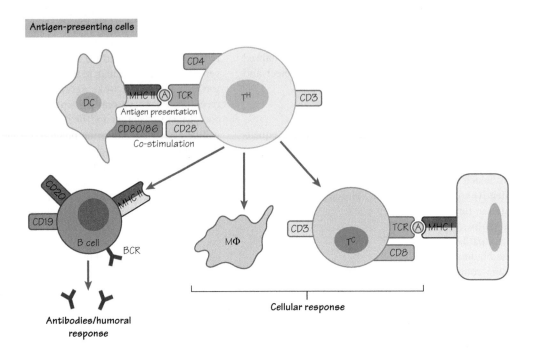

Antigen-presenting cells

Antigen presentation

Co-stimulation

Cellular response

Antibodies/humoral response

(b) Antigen presentation in transplantation

Indirect antigen presentation

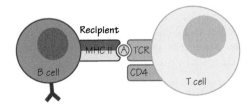

- Peptide derived from a donor protein
- Recipient HLA molecule (or the same HLA as the recipient)

Direct antigen presentation

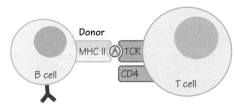

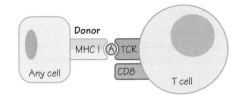

- Peptide derived from donor or recipient protein
- Donor HLA molecule
- 5–10% of ALL circulating T cells may recognise allo-MHC via the direct pathway

Transplantation at a Glance, First Edition. Menna Clatworthy, Christopher Watson, Michael Allison and John Dark.

The adaptive immune system

The adaptive immune system is more specific than the innate system, and can amplify and increase the specificity of the immune response. The main protagonists are antigen-presenting cells (APCs), B cells and T cells. Each of these cell types has a different function and can be identified by the expression of a number of specific surface molecules which have been designated with CD (cluster of differentiation) numbers. Thus, B cells can be identified by the expression of CD19 and CD20, and T cells by the expression of CD2 and CD3.

The adaptive immune response has two arms, the humoral arm (antibody-mediated) and the cellular arm (principally mediated by cytotoxic T cells [T^C], which express the molecule CD8). At the centre of both arms are T helper cells (T^H), which express CD4.

CD4 T cells can be activated only when they 'see' peptide antigen displayed in the groove of a specific family of glycoproteins, the major histocompatibility complex (MHC) class II molecules (also known as human leucocyte antigens [HLAs]). Each CD4 T cell has a unique T cell receptor (TCR), which allows it to recognise a specific peptide-MHC II complex, and CD4 acts as a co-receptor to stabilise the interaction between TCR and MHC. The expression of MHC class II molecules is limited to three main cell types, which are known as professional APCs:

1. Dendritic cells (DCs)
2. B cells
3. Macrophages (less efficient APCs).

These APCs have the ability to internalise protein antigens present outside of the cell. APCs have different sorts of receptors, which allow them to internalise antigen. B cells bind antigen via their B cell receptor (BCR), which is specific for that particular antigen. In contrast, DCs and macrophages internalise molecules via a number of receptors that are not antigen-specific, for example FcγRs or complement receptors. They can also internalise antigen via endocytosis.

Once internalised, these antigens are then processed within intracellular compartments (endosomes or lysosomes) and degraded into peptides. The endosome fuses with an exosome containing MHC class II molecules (derived from the golgi body of the cell). Peptides are subsequently loaded into the groove of specific class II molecules into which they specifically fit. Peptide-loaded class II molecules are then transported to the surface of the cell where they are accessible to CD4 T cells.

In addition to presenting antigen to CD4 T cells, APCs also provide co-stimulatory signals to allow full activation (*see* Chapter 9). This involves the interaction of pairs of molecules, one found on the surface of the T cell and the other on the APC.

T cell ligand	Co-stimulatory molecule on APC
CD28	CD80 (B7.1)
CD28	CD86 (B7.2)
CD40L (CD154)	CD40
ICOS	ICOSL (CD275)

Once a CD4 T cell is activated, it may provide help to B cells through the production of cytokines (principally IL-4) and through contact-dependent signals, initiating a humoral response. Thus, the interaction between a B cell and a T cell is a two-way process of mutual help and activation. Alternatively, CD4 T cells may provide help to CD8 T cells and macrophages via the production of a different set of cytokines (principally interferon-γ), initiating a cellular response.

CD8 T cells can only be activated when they 'see' peptide antigen displayed in the groove of an MHC class I molecule. Each CD8 T cell has a unique TCR, which allows it to recognise a specific peptide-MHC I complex. Almost all cell types express MHC class I molecules. In contrast to MHC class II molecules, the antigens displayed on class I molecules are not obtained from outside the cell, but rather from the cytoplasm of the cell. Thus, in the case of a viral infection, viral antigen samples from the cytoplasm will be processed, loaded onto class I molecules and sent to the surface of the cell to allow detection by CD8 T cells.

Antigen presentation in transplantation

In transplantation, direct and indirect alloantigen presentation occur. These can be defined as follows.

• *Direct antigen presentation* – donor antigen is presented on donor MHC class I or class II molecule. Between 5 and 10% of the recipient's T cell repertoire may recognise foreign MHC, therefore this form of antigen presentation is very important in initiating transplant rejection.
• *Indirect antigen presentation* – donor antigen is presented on recipient MHC class II molecule, which has been processed by the recipient APC in the conventional way.

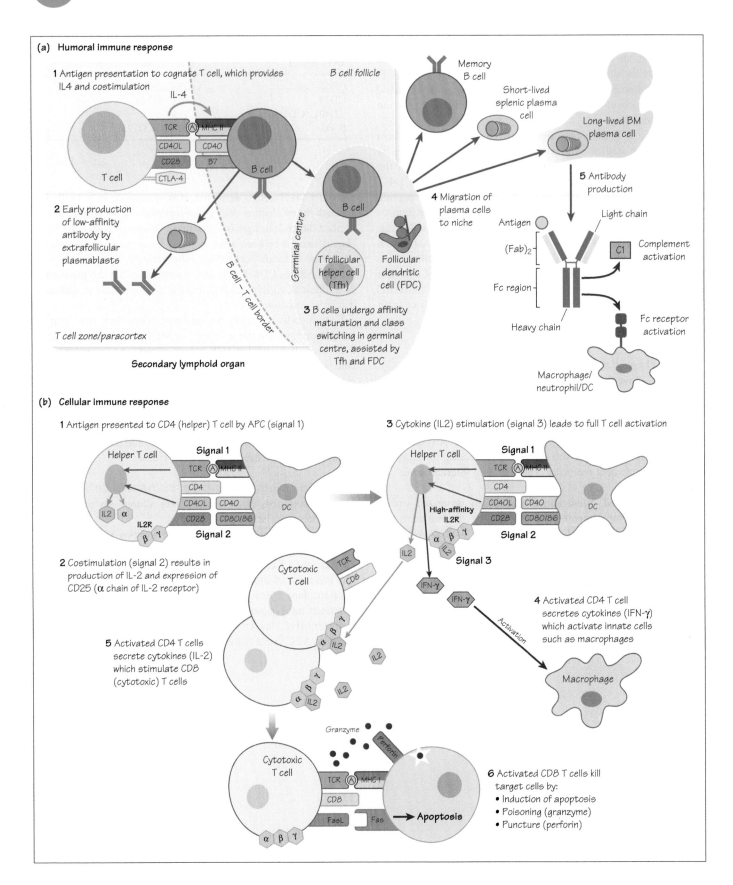

Humoral (antibody-mediated) immunity

Antibodies (also known as immunoglobulins, Ig) are produced by terminally differentiated B cells, known as plasma cells. Antibody responses to protein antigens require T cell help (T-dependent antigens). The production of antibodies to carbohydrate antigens (e.g. the polysaccharide capsule surrounding some bacteria) occurs in the marginal zone of the spleen, and does not require T cell help (T-independent responses). In transplantation, T-dependent responses are the most important and occur via the following steps.

(1.) B cells recognise antigen via their surface B cell receptor (BCR), a membrane-bound IgM antibody molecule. BCR-bound antigen is internalised, processed and presented on the surface of the B cell in the groove of class II major histocompatibility (MHC) molecules, also known as human leucocyte antigens (HLA). The antigen is presented to a 'cognate' T cell, i.e. one that has a cell surface receptor (the T cell receptor [TCR]), which recognises the same antigen in the context of that particular MHC molecule. As the B cell presents antigen, it also provides a co-stimulatory signal to the T cell. This occurs by the interaction of pairs of molecules found on the surface of B and T cells (e.g. CD86 on B cells and CD28 on T cells). The T cell in turn provides help to the B cell, including the provision of the cytokine interleukin (IL)-4.

(2.) Following the receipt of T cell help, some B cells proliferate and form short-lived plasmablasts, which produce large quantities of low-affinity antibody.

(3.) Other B cells move into B cell follicles in lymphoid tissue and subsequently undergo class switching (they begin to express IgG or IgE rather than IgM) and affinity maturation in the germinal centre. Affinity maturation involves the introduction of mutations into the genes encoding the variable (antigen-binding) region of the antibody (somatic hypermutation) to generate a BCR with higher affinity for antigen.

(4.) Following affinity maturation in the germinal centre, some B cells become 'memory' B cells (characterised by surface expression of CD27). They continually circulate through the secondary lymphoid organs and if the individual is re-challenged with an antigen, these memory B cells obtain cognate T cell help and rapidly proliferate to produce large quantities of low-affinity antibody. Other germinal centre B cells form short-lived plasmablasts, producing a temporary burst of antibody. A minority of plasma cells migrate from the spleen and lymph nodes to niches within bone marrow.

(5.) Bone marrow plasma cells are long-lived and reside in their niches for prolonged periods (probably decades or even the entire lifespan of the human). These plasma cells do not proliferate (and are therefore difficult to target therapeutically), but exist as 'protein factories' producing serum IgG.

Antibodies (or immunoglobulins) are comprised of a heavy chain and a light chain, and the former determines the antibody class, for example, IgG antibodies have a γ heavy chain. Immunoglobulins have a variable antigen-binding F(ab)2 region and an Fc region responsible for mediating many effector functions of antibody via complement activation and Fc receptor binding. Antibodies mediate their effector function by directly neutralising pathogen-related toxins, opsonising pathogens for uptake by Fc receptors or flagging cells for antibody-dependent cellular cytotoxicity (ADCC).

Cellular immunity

The effector function of the cellular immune response is principally mediated by cytotoxic (CD8) T cells. As their name suggests, they are professional cell killers that can poison cells (by secretion of granzyme), punch holes in the cell membrane (using perforin) or induce the cell to commit suicide (apoptosis) via the Fas-FasL pathway. CD8 T cells have TCRs that recognise peptides processed from intracellular proteins (e.g. viral proteins) and presented on the surface in the groove of MHC class I molecules. In addition, cytokine help for CD8 T cells is provided by CD4 T cells, in the form of IL-2. In order for CD4 T cells to be activated, they must have antigen presented to them on MHC class II molecules by APCs (*see* Chapter 8), which is recognised by the TCR (signal 1). A co-stimulatory signal is also required (signal 2). APCs up-regulate expression of co-stimulatory molecules when they detect a danger signal, for example a pathogen-associated molecular pattern (PAMP). If signal 1 is received in the absence of signal 2, then the T cell will become anergic or will undergo apoptosis. This acts as a means of guarding against activating CD4 T cells against self-antigens. If both signals 1 and 2 are received then the CD4 T cell will up-regulate expression of CD25 (the α-chain of the IL2 receptor [IL2R]), converting it from its low-affinity dimeric form to a high-affinity trimeric form, which avidly binds IL2 providing a further activation signal to the T cell (signal 3). The CD4 T cell will then proliferate, synthesise IL-2 (stimulating self-activation and the activation of CD8 T cells) and begin to orchestrate a powerful adaptive immune response. Following this process, some CD4 and CD8 T cells become memory cells, and can be more readily activated following subsequent exposure to the same antigen.

CD4 T cells can also provide help to activate macrophages through the production of cytokines such as interferon-γ (IFN- γ). In response to IFN- γ, macrophages (and dendritic cells) produce IL12, which further drives the production of IFN- γ by T cells. Helper T cells programmed or polarised to produce IL-2 and IFN-γ are known as Th1 cells, and this lineage is characterised by the expression of the transcription factor Tbet. Those producing IL4 and promoting humoral immunity are known as Th2 cells, and are characterised by expression of GATA3. More recently, CD4 T cells that produce IL17 have been described (Th17 cells). IL17 plays a pathogenic role in a number of autoimmune diseases, although its role in transplant rejection is less clear.

Regulatory immune cells

Some T and B cells have the capacity to inhibit immune activation and play an important role in limiting pathogenic autoimmune responses. Regulatory T cells are characterised by the expression of the transcription factor foxp3 and have high surface expression of CD4 and CD25. They mediate suppression principally through the production of transforming growth factor (TGF)-β and IL10.

Regulatory B cells are CD19+, CD24 high and CD38 high, and they mediate immune suppression by production of IL-10. These cells may potentially play an important role in the induction of transplant tolerance.

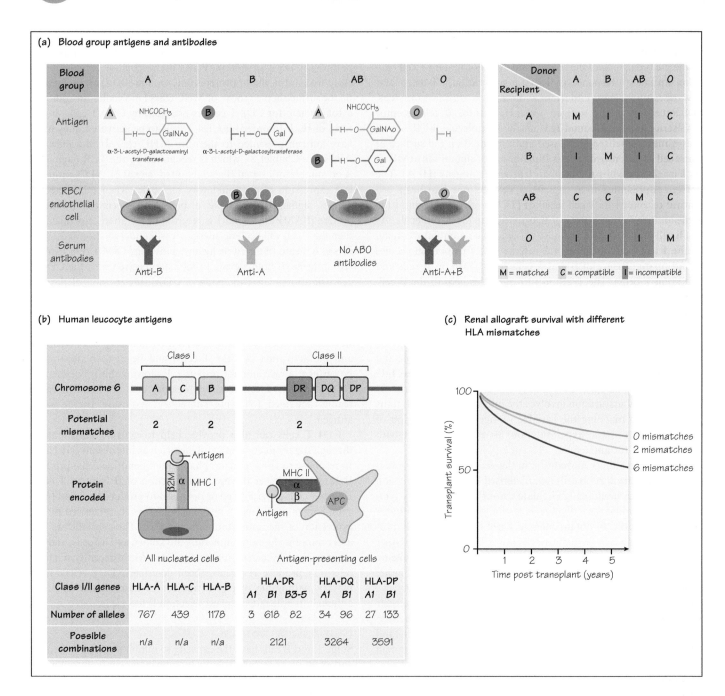

Tissue typing of transplant recipients is required to assess their immunological profile in order to find an optimally matched organ. This involves identifying their ABO blood group, and determining which human leucocyte antigens (HLAs) their cells express. These tests are performed as part of the transplant assessment process, well in advance of the actual transplant.

ABO antigens

ABO antigens are carbohydrate molecules found on the surface of red blood cells and endothelial cells. Group O individuals (who

lack A and B antigens) develop antibodies to both A and B antigens. This is thought to be driven by cross-reactivity with microbial antigens. In group A individuals, B antibodies are present, while group B individuals have A antibodies. AB individuals have no A or B antibodies. Transplantation of an organ into an ABO-incompatible recipient, e.g. an organ from a group A donor into a group O recipient, would lead to immediate binding of A antibodies to graft endothelium, and to hyperacute rejection. Thus, the first step of tissue typing is to ascertain the recipient's blood group so that an ABO-compatible donor can

Transplantation at a Glance, First Edition. Menna Clatworthy, Christopher Watson, Michael Allison and John Dark.

be selected. There are two methods used to perform ABO typing.

1 Forward typing – the recipient's erythrocytes are mixed with anti-A or anti-B serum. If the erythrocytes express A antigens, then agglutination of the cells will occur when incubated with anti-A serum, etc.

2 Reverse typing – the recipient's serum is mixed with erythrocytes of known ABO type. This test is used to confirm the results of forward typing. It can also be used to determine the quantity of ABO antibodies present by performing serial dilutions of the recipient's serum prior to incubation with erythrocytes. The ABO titre gives a measure of the concentration of ABO antibodies, and is quantified as the final dilution at which agglutination takes place, e.g. 1 in 32. The latter test is used in preparation for ABO-incompatible transplantation to assess the requirement for antibody removal during desensitisation (*see* Chapter 12).

HLA antigens

The human leucocyte antigens (HLA), also known as the major histocompatibility complex (MHC) molecules, are a family of highly polymorphic glycoproteins found on the surface of cells. They are divided into class I and class II molecules. Class I molecules are found on the surface of all nucleated cells and are composed of a polymorphic α chain combined with an invariant subunit (β2 microglobulin). Intracellular protein antigens are processed and presented on class I molecules to CD8 T cells (*see* Chapter 8). Class II molecules are found only on the surface of antigen-presenting cells (APCs) and are composed of two highly polymorphic subunits, an α-chain and a β-chain. APCs internalise extracellular antigens, process them and load peptides onto class II molecules for presentation to CD4 T cells (*see* Chapters 8 and 9).

HLAs are encoded by a cluster of genes on chromosome 6. In humans, there are 3 HLA class I genes (A, B and C). These genes are extremely variable, and encode highly polymorphic α-chains. More than 700 variants of the A gene, 1000 variants of the B gene and 400 variants of the C gene have been identified. This variation makes it unlikely that an unrelated donor and recipient will have exactly the same HLA antigen on the surface of their cells. Such extensive genetic variability is unusual in the human genome and is thought to have arisen as a strategy to prevent a single viral mutation (which might prevent viral peptide being loaded onto class I molecules) from conferring virulence against all humans, as there would likely be a class I variant in some individuals in the population which could present the mutated viral peptide.

The HLA class II genes (DP, DQ and DR) are also found on chromosome 6, and are more complex than the class I genes.

HLA-DP is encoded by a polymorphic α-chain gene (HLA-DPA1; >25 different alleles described) and a polymorphic β-chain (HLA-DPB1; >130 alleles described).

HLA-DQ is encoded by a polymorphic α-chain gene (HLA-DQA1; >30 alleles described) and a polymorphic β-chain (HLA-DQB1; >90 alleles described).

HLA-DR is encoded by a polymorphic α-chain gene (HLA-DRA; three alleles described) and four highly polymorphic β-chain genes (HLA-DRB1, B3, B4 and B5; >600 variants described). The DRB1 gene encodes the β-chain of the classical DR class II molecule. The most commonly observed DR antigen in UK donors (arising from variants of the DRB1-β and DRα genes) is the DR4 antigen (present in 35% of donors). The DRB3, 4 and 5 genes also encode β-chains that can complex with the DR α-chain, and give rise to the HLA-DR52, 53 and 51 antigens respectively.

HLA nomenclature

Two parallel systems of nomenclature are applied to HLA antigens.

1 *Serological* – this was the initial system used to name HLA antigens based on their reactivity to standardised antisera. In transplantation, 55 HLA-A, B and DR antigens are defined based on reactivity to a set of broad antisera. Some of these antigens can be subdivided using more specific antisera (e.g. HLA-A10 can be split into HLA-A25(10) and HLA-A26(10)).

2 *DNA sequence* – advances in molecular biology have allowed the specific sequences of different HLA genes to be determined. Allele names are prefixed with a '*'; for example, the alleles encoding the HLA-A3 antigen are named A*03. Different A3 alleles are then given different numbers, e.g. A*0301, A*0302, etc.

In clinical practice in solid organ transplantation, HLA type is now determined by DNA sequencing.

HLA matching

Given that an individual has two copies of each HLA gene, the maximum number of mismatches that can occur between a donor and recipient is 12, i.e. two A mismatches, two B mismatches, etc. However, in renal transplantation only A, B and DR mismatches are considered, so the maximum number of mismatches possible is six. Such a mismatch would be described as a 2-2-2 mismatch (2 A, 2 B and 2 DR mismatches). The best mismatch would be a 0-0-0 mismatch. The more mismatches that are present, the more likely that the allograft will be recognised as foreign and rejected. This is reflected in allograft survival data which suggest that 80% of those patients receiving a 0-0-0 mismatched kidney will still have a functioning allograft at 5 years compared with 60% of those receiving a 2-2-2 mismatched kidney. DR mismatches are more significant than A or B mismatches, therefore every effort is made to avoid DR mismatches.

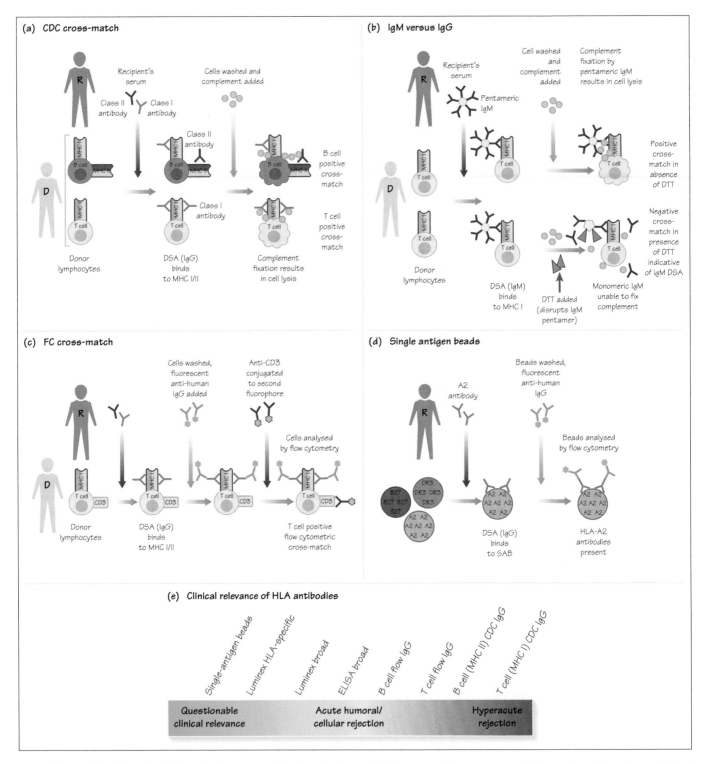

In addition to identifying the HLA antigens expressed by the recipient, it is also important to determine whether the recipient has any circulating HLA antibodies, as the presence of donor-specific HLA antibodies at the time of transplantation may result in hyperacute rejection and loss of the graft. Testing for HLA antibodies occurs both prior to and at the time of transplantation, as follows:

1 *During transplant assessment/while on the waiting list* – recipient serum is screened for the presence of HLA antibodies using a number of techniques with varying sensitivity.

2 *At the time of the transplantation* – a cross-match test is performed to make absolutely sure that the recipient does not have any donor-reactive antibodies.

Transplantation at a Glance, First Edition. Menna Clatworthy, Christopher Watson, Michael Allison and John Dark.

Screening prior to transplantation

Solid phase assays

ELISA-based assays – ELISA (enzyme-linked immunosorbent assay) is performed by coating the wells of a multi-well plate with purified HLA antigens. The recipient's serum is placed in these wells, incubated, washed and detected using a labelled anti-human IgG antibody. This technique is more sensitive than complement-dependent cytotoxicity (CDC) and allows the identification of non-complement-fixing antibodies.

Flow cytometric/luminex assays – the recipient's serum is incubated with fluorescent beads that have been pre-coated with HLA antigens. A secondary anti-human IgG antibody labelled with a different fluorescent colour is added to identify beads with antibody bound, and the sample analysed by flow cytometry. This assay is even more sensitive than ELISA-based techniques.

Calculated reaction frequency (cRF)

Having defined what HLA-specific antibodies are in the recipient's serum, the reaction frequency is calculated. This is the proportion of a pool of 10,000 blood group-identical organ donors against which the recipient has HLA antibodies. A recipient is considered to be highly sensitised if they have a cRF ≥85%, implying that they will be incompatible with more than 85% of all blood group-identical organ donors.

The cRF has replaced panel reactive antibodies (PRA) as a measure of sensitisation. PRA was defined as the proportion of an arbitrarily defined collection of lymphocytes (the panel) that underwent lysis when recipient sera and rabbit complement were added. Hence the PRA test identifies only complement-fixing antibodies and has low sensitivity.

Screening at the time of transplantation

Cross-matching is used to identify the presence of complement-fixing, donor-reactive HLA-antibodies in the recipient's serum.

Cytotoxic (CDC) cross-match

A cytotoxic cross-match is performed by incubating the recipient's serum with donor T cells (expressing MHC class I antigens) and donor B cells (expressing both MHC class I and class II antigens) and complement. These B and T cells are usually obtained from donor lymph nodes or spleen. If antibodies are present in the recipient's serum, they will bind to donor cells, activate complement, and cause lysis of donor cells by CDC. If T and B cells are lysed, this indicates the presence of class I +/– class II antibodies. If B cells alone are lysed it is indicative of the presence of MHC class II antibodies, or a non-HLA binding antibody.

IgM and IgG donor-specific antibodies can be distinguished by performing the cross-match in the presence or absence of dithiothreitol (DTT). DTT disaggregates multimeric IgM. Thus, a CDC cross-match that is positive in the absence of DTT but negative in the presence of DTT suggests the presence of donor-specific IgM antibodies, which do not represent a significant risk to the allograft.

A positive T cell CDC cross-match resulting from an IgM antibody is not a contraindication to transplantation. In contrast, a positive T cell CDC cross-match due to an IgG antibody precludes transplantation and, should the transplant proceed, would likely result in hyperacute rejection.

The importance of a positive B cell CDC cross-match in the absence of a positive T cell CDC cross-match is less clear and must be interpreted in the light of HLA antibody screening performed prior to transplantation. If the recipient is known to have MHC class II antibodies, then a B cell CDC cross-match is likely due to a complement-fixing class II antibody. Both endothelial cells and renal tubular cells may express class II antigens, particularly during inflammation, thus the presence of such antibodies should be considered to be a contraindication to transplantation. Most class II antibodies are directed against HLA-DR antigens. HLA-DP and DQ antibodies occur less frequently, and may be variably pathogenic.

If a recipient is non-sensitised, and has no known donor-specific antibodies (DSA), then an isolated positive B cell CDC is unlikely to be due to a class II antibody, but may still indicate the presence of a pathogenic antibody or autoantibody. B cells express surface monomeric IgM (their B cell receptor) and also an Fcγ receptor (FcγRIIB), both of which may bind non-HLA antibodies, which are usually autoantibodies. Historically, non-HLA antibodies were considered not to be harmful to the graft; however, there is increasing evidence that they may have a deleterious effect on long-term graft function and survival.

Flow cytometric cross-match

CDC cross-match testing is effective in identifying the presence of antibodies that would result in hyperacute rejection, but is not sufficiently sensitive to identify all DSA. Some IgG isotypes do not fix complement efficiently (e.g. IgG4) and will therefore not be detected by a CDC cross-match, but might still damage the graft by activating phagocytes via FcγRs. Flow cytometric cross-matching overcomes these limitations. It involves incubating donor lymphocytes and recipient serum in the absence of complement, and applying a fluorescently labelled secondary anti-human IgG antibody to identify the presence of IgG bound to lymphocytes by flow cytometry. This amplification step increases the sensitivity of the test compared with CDC cross-matching. Cells are also incubated with fluorescently labelled antibodies recognising B and T cells (e.g. anti-CD19 and CD3 antibodies respectively). Thus, IgG antibodies binding T and/or B cells can be distinguished.

A positive T cell 'flow' cross-match in the presence of a negative CDC cross-match usually reflects the presence of a lower titre of MHC class I-binding DSA. Alternatively, it may indicate the presence of a non-complement-fixing IgG isotype. In such cases, the antibody may not be sufficient to mediate hyperacute rejection, but can cause early antibody-mediated rejection (AMR) and would also be considered a contraindication to transplantation.

The information obtained from antibody screening and the cross-match allow an assessment of the risk of humoral alloreactivity.

Transplantation without a cross-match

The cross-match is time-consuming and increases cold ischaemic times. In selected patients it may be safe to proceed to transplantation without performing a cross-match. Such patients:

- are receiving their first transplant;
- have no history of sensitising events, such as blood transfusions or pregnancies;
- have no detectable HLA antibodies.

In such patients, the probability of a positive cross-match is extremely low. The application of this strategy is dependent on having up-to-date information about the HLA antibody status of recipients, and thus requires potential recipients to be regularly screened for antibodies, e.g. once every 3 months.

12 Antibody-incompatible transplantation

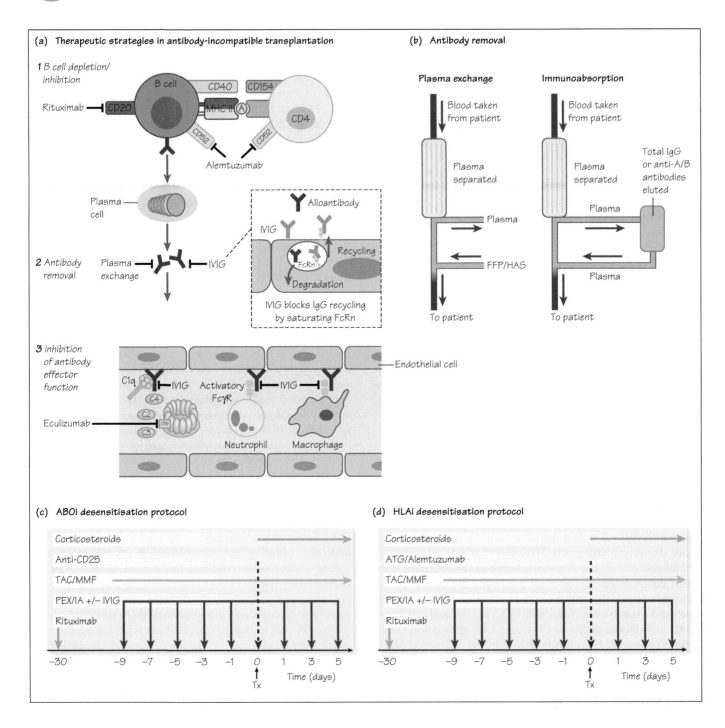

(a) Therapeutic strategies in antibody-incompatible transplantation

1 B cell depletion/inhibition

Rituximab ⊣ CD20

B cell — CD40 — CD154 — CD4 — MHC II (A)

Alemtuzumab ⊣ CD52

Plasma cell

2 Antibody removal — Plasma exchange ⊣ IVIG

Alloantibody

IVIG — FcRn — Recycling — Degradation

IVIG blocks IgG recycling by saturating FcRn

3 Inhibition of antibody effector function

C1q — C4 — C2 — C3 — C5b

Eculizumab ⊣

IVIG — Activatory FcγR — IVIG

Endothelial cell

Neutrophil — Macrophage

(b) Antibody removal

Plasma exchange

Blood taken from patient → Plasma separated → Plasma → FFP/HAS → To patient

Immunoabsorption

Blood taken from patient → Plasma separated → Plasma → Total IgG or anti-A/B antibodies eluted → Plasma → To patient

(c) ABOi desensitisation protocol

Corticosteroids
Anti-CD25
TAC/MMF
PEX/IA +/− IVIG
Rituximab

-30 … -9 -7 -5 -3 -1 0 1 3 5   Time (days)
Tx

(d) HLAi desensitisation protocol

Corticosteroids
ATG/Alemtuzumab
TAC/MMF
PEX/IA +/− IVIG
Rituximab

-30 … -9 -7 -5 -3 -1 0 1 3 5   Time (days)
Tx

An ever-increasing number of patients on the transplant waiting list and a static rate of DBD donation has forced the development of DCD donor programmes and the increasing use of living donors. If a patient has a potential living donor, one of the major barriers to successful transplantation is donor–recipient immunological incompatibility, i.e. the presence of circulating donor-specific ABO or HLA antibodies. In such cases, transplantation in the absence of antibody removal would result in hyperacute rejection and immediate loss of the graft (*see* Chapter 28). Even low levels of antibody can cause acute antibody-mediated rejection (AMR), which has a poor prognosis.

Antibody specificity
ABO antibodies
ABO antigens are not only found on the surface of red blood cells, but also on endothelial cells (*see* Chapter 10). ABO antigens are carbohydrates (not protein antigens, in contrast to HLA). Carbohydrate antigens are termed 'T-independent' antigens, i.e. B cells

Transplantation at a Glance, First Edition. Menna Clatworthy, Christopher Watson, Michael Allison and John Dark.

do not require T cell help to make antibodies to such antigens. B cells in the marginal zone of the spleen are important for T-independent antibody responses.

Group O individuals (who lack A and B antigens), develop antibodies to both antigens. This is thought to be driven by cross-reactivity with microbial antigens. In group A individuals, B antibodies are present, while group B individuals have A antibodies. Thirty per cent of potential living donor-recipients have ABO-incompatible (ABOi) donors (mainly group O recipients with donors who are A, B or AB to whom they have antibodies).

HLA antibodies

One-third of patients on the transplant waiting list have detectable antibodies to human leucocyte antigens (HLA). These patients are termed 'sensitised'. HLA molecules are highly polymorphic (see Chapter 10), so if the immune system encounters foreign cells expressing HLA molecules, they will likely be different from self-HLA and will induce an immune response. There are three common scenarios in which non-self HLA has been encountered by patients awaiting transplantation, termed as 'sensitising events':
• blood transfusion
• pregnancy
• previous transplantation (including skin grafts).
These sensitising events may result in the formation of antibodies to multiple HLA molecules, both MHC class I and class II.

Desensitisation procedure

A number of strategies are used to facilitate antibody incompatible transplantation including:
• removal of donor-specific antibodies (DSA) to a 'safe' level prior to transplantation
• prevention of the synthesis of further DSA, by inhibiting memory B and T cells, and plasma cells
• inhibition of antibody-mediated complement activation.

Antibody removal

This involves filtration or plasma exchange; the patient's blood is passed through a special column that removes the antibody component. Antibody removal may be more or less specific, for example there are columns that bind only anti-A and anti-B antibodies, and do not deplete the patient's general pool of IgG (Glycosorb columns). Some systems return the patient's filtered plasma, while others require replacement with human albumin solution (HAS) or fresh frozen plasma (FFP). Most centres will begin antibody removal in the week prior to the planned transplantation, since the number of sessions required varies, depending on the starting titre of DSA. Intravenous immunoglobulin (pooled human IgG, IVIG) can also reduce DSA through blockade of FcRn, the receptor responsible for recycling IgG.

Prevention of the formation of additional DSA

IgG is produced by plasma cells, which are generated from B cells following the receipt of T cell help in the germinal centres of lymph nodes and spleen. The emerging plasma cells migrate from these organs to niches within bone marrow, where they reside for prolonged periods. Long-lived plasma cells do not proliferate (and are therefore difficult to target therapeutically), but exist as 'protein factories' producing 95% of serum IgG. Some post-germinal centre B cells become 'memory' B cells (characterised by surface expression of CD27). They continually circulate through the secondary lymphoid organs and if the individual is re-challenged with an antigen, these memory B cells can rapidly proliferate to produce large quantities of low-affinity antibody. Thus, to prevent re-accumulation of DSA post transplant, a strategy that targets B cells, T cells and plasma cells is required.

Most centres will start immunosuppression some time before antibody removal begins. This involves the administration of a lymphocyte-depleting agent, the nature of which varies from centre to centre. Some centres use pan-lymphocyte depletion with anti-thymocyte globulin (ATG) or alemtuzumab (CamPath-1H), while others use B cell-targeted therapy, such as the CD20 monoclonal antibody rituximab. Early attempts at antibody-incompatible transplantation utilised splenectomy as a means of depleting B cells. Each of the above agents has its own merits and disadvantages: ATG is a polyclonal mixture of antibodies that targets both B and T cells. On the negative side it is a profound immunosuppressant and is associated with an increased risk of infection. Alemtuzumab, an anti-CD52 antibody, depletes B cells, T cells, DCs and natural killer cells. It appears to have a relatively good safety profile in terms of infection. Often the choice of agent will depend on the perceived magnitude of the donor-specific immune response.

The proteosome inhibitor bortezomib has also been used to target plasma cells in transplantation, but is currently an experimental treatment only.

ABO-incompatible transplantation is more amenable to desensitisation procedures, with patient and allograft survival nearing that of ABO-compatible living donor transplants in experienced centres. HLA-incompatible transplantation appears to pose a greater challenge, and even with desensitisation, some patients' DSA titres do not fall sufficiently to allow safe transplantation.

Prevention of complement activation

IgG immune complexes activate complement via the classical pathway. This generates the C3 convertase C4b2b, which catalyses the conversion of C3 to C3a. This in turn activates C5 and initiates the formation of the membrane attack complex (MAC) which disrupts cell membrane integrity, leading to cell lysis. A monoclonal antibody, eculizumab, specifically binds to C5a and inhibits its activity, preventing MAC formation. Early studies suggest that this agent may well be of use post-transplant in preventing the deleterious effects of antibody-mediated complement activation. IVIG may also act to block FcγR-mediated activation of phagocytes.

Paired exchange kidney donation

Patients with a potential antibody-incompatible donor can be placed into a national pool with other antibody-incompatible donor–recipient pairs. Attempts are made to match one pair with another such that an antibody-compatible transplant may occur, i.e. the donor from pair A is compatible with the recipient from pair B and vice versa. More complex exchanges between three or more pairs are possible. Such kidney exchanges allow transplantation to proceed while avoiding the rigors of desensitisation.

13 Organ allocation

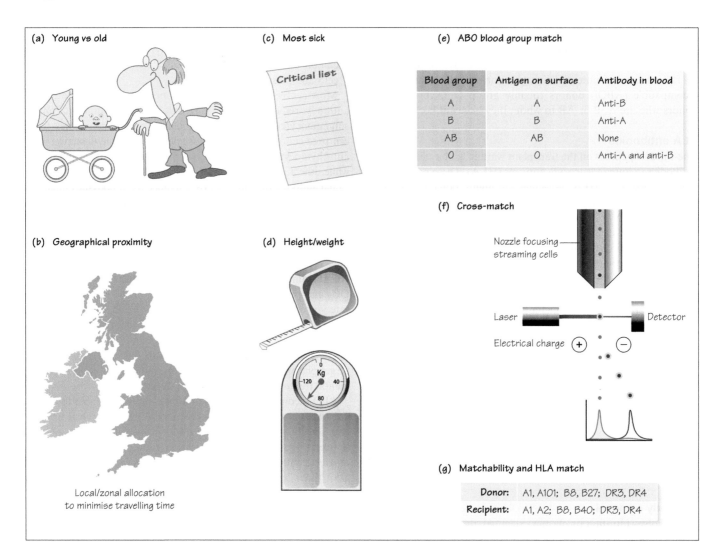

(a) Young vs old

(b) Geographical proximity

Local/zonal allocation to minimise travelling time

(c) Most sick

Critical list

(d) Height/weight

Kg

(e) ABO blood group match

Blood group	Antigen on surface	Antibody in blood
A	A	Anti-B
B	B	Anti-A
AB	AB	None
O	O	Anti-A and anti-B

(f) Cross-match

Nozzle focusing streaming cells

Laser — Detector

Electrical charge (+) (−)

(g) Matchability and HLA match

Donor:	A1, A101; B8, B27; DR3, DR4
Recipient:	A1, A2; B8, B40; DR3, DR4

There are many more people on the transplant waiting list than there are organs available. To manage this shortage access to the waiting list is restricted to those meeting strict eligibility rules. Once on the waiting list allocation follows pre-defined rules to ensure fairness.

Eligibility for transplantation

Criteria vary from organ to organ, and country to country. In addition, different considerations may be necessary for patients needing a second transplant after the first has failed, particularly since for most organs the results for second and subsequent transplants are inferior to first transplants. For kidney, pancreas and liver there must be an expectation that the recipient will survive 5 years after the operation. UK listing criteria are given below.

Kidney transplantation

Already on, or estimated to be within 6 months of starting dialysis (e.g. using a reciprocal creatinine graph). Re-transplantation is permitted providing it is surgically feasible and the patient is fit; the main limiting factor is sensitisation against HLA antigens.

Pancreas transplantation

1 *Combined (simultaneous) pancreas and kidney (SPK) transplantation*: GFR ≤ 20 ml/min or on dialysis **and** type 1 diabetes (or type 2 if BMI <30 kg/m^2).

2 *Pancreas or islet transplantation alone (PTA/ITA)*: life-threatening hypoglycaemic unawareness.

3 *Pancreas after kidney transplantation (PAK)*: severe diabetic complications and satisfactory function of prior renal transplant, since function is affected by increased doses of nephrotoxic immunosuppression.

Liver transplantation

There is no bar on re-transplantation, but since results of re-transplants are so much poorer, the patient should be otherwise in good health. Individual criteria exist for subgroups, such as hepatocellular tumours or acute liver failure (*see* Chapter 33).

Transplantation at a Glance, First Edition. Menna Clatworthy, Christopher Watson, Michael Allison and John Dark.

Heart transplantation

Patients are accepted according to internationally agreed criteria. Many patients are now supported by mechanical devices, and are regarded as stable on the waiting list. They only receive priority if they develop complications such as drive-line infections. Re-transplants can be done with reasonably good outcomes, but not in the first 3 months after the initial procedure.

Lung transplantation

Most patients are now listed for bilateral lung transplants. The only group regularly receiving single lungs are those with fibrotic disease, where the shrunken chest cavity cannot easily accept a pair of lungs.

Re-transplants are done with increasing frequency, although still amount to only 5–6% of activity.

Principles in organ allocation

Organ allocation is an exercise in distributive justice, how to fairly divide up a limited resource. There are several criteria that may be used for organ allocation.

Equity (fairness): everyone should have equal access to organs. Such a scheme would allocate organs first to those who have been waiting longest, and to young and old alike.

Utility: organs should be allocated to achieve the greatest number of life-years following transplantation, independent of other factors. For example, since outcomes of kidney transplantation are poorer in those already on dialysis and in the elderly, these two groups would be excluded in a utilitarian allocation scheme, in direct contrast to the egalitarian approach.

Greatest need: the organ goes to the person whose medical condition demands it the most.

Greatest benefit: organs are allocated to achieve the greatest benefit, in terms of life-years gained, compared with remaining on the waiting list. Such allocation acknowledges that organs are different, with young donor organs having a better anticipated longevity than older organs. Thus an old donor kidney may be best allocated to an older recipient, who has a high mortality on dialysis and for whom an old kidney would increase their survival significantly. A young recipient has a better survival on dialysis so there is less gain from having an old kidney, which would last only a short time period.

Allocation in practice

In reality, current allocation schemes involve a mixture of the above principles. Organs are allocated to ABO-identical recipients, with the exception of group A organs, which may go to AB recipients, and occasional group O organs, which may go to group B (or A or AB) recipients in special circumstances (e.g. medical urgency or HLA sensitisation).

Organs are transplanted to avoid pre-existing donor-specific HLA antibodies (a positive cross-match), with the exception of the liver, which can be transplanted into a recipient who possesses antibodies to the donor's MHC class 1 antigens.

Kidney

Kidneys are allocated primarily to HLA-matched recipients, prioritising sensitised patients over non-sensitised, children over

adults. Thereafter allocation is according to a complex formula that assigns points for:
- HLA mismatch, aiming to optimise matching
- time on the waiting list, prioritising long waiters
- sensitisation (HLA antibodies) and matchibility (unusual HLA type), giving priority to patients who are hardest to find a compatible transplant
- HLA-B and -DR homozygous recipients, correcting an imbalance that prioritising according to HLA mismatch creates
- age difference, aiming to minimise age difference between donor and recipient.

In addition children (under 18) get priority over adults.

Pancreas for islets or whole organ

An algorithm assigns points for:
- HLA mismatch, aiming to optimise matching
- HLA sensitisation and matchibility
- waiting time, giving additional priority to an islet recipient awaiting a second graft and a pancreas recipient on dialysis
- distance of donor to recipient centre, to minimise ischaemic time.

Liver

Livers are allocated within seven zones in the UK corresponding to each liver transplant unit. Priority is given to the sickest patient (UKELD score, *see* Chapter 33) of a compatible size – big livers don't fit small abdomens.

A 'super-urgent' scheme exists for anyone with acute liver failure with an expected of survival of less than 3 days; a third of these patients die while waiting and outcomes are poorer than for chronic liver disease.

Heart

Like livers, hearts and lungs are allocated within zones corresponding to each of the six transplant centres. Matching is done by blood group and size of donor, which needs to be within 10% of that of the recipient. Female hearts placed in male recipients do measurably less well, and this combination is avoided.

There is also an urgent scheme for hearts, which accounts for nearly half of all transplants performed. The results are at least as good as those for 'elective' patients. These recipients have the most to gain from transplantation.

Lung

Size is of great importance in lung allocation – large lungs do not fit into small recipients. If small lungs are placed in a large chest they become over-inflated. Allocation is done as for hearts and livers, on a local basis, but there is no urgent system. Individual centres identify the sickest patients on their waiting list. A lung that cannot be used locally is offered nationally around the other centres.

Intestine

Intestinal donors are offered as a priority to the four intestinal transplant centres (two adult, two child). For most intestinal transplants size is the critical factor, with only the smaller donors (below 50 kg) being suitable.

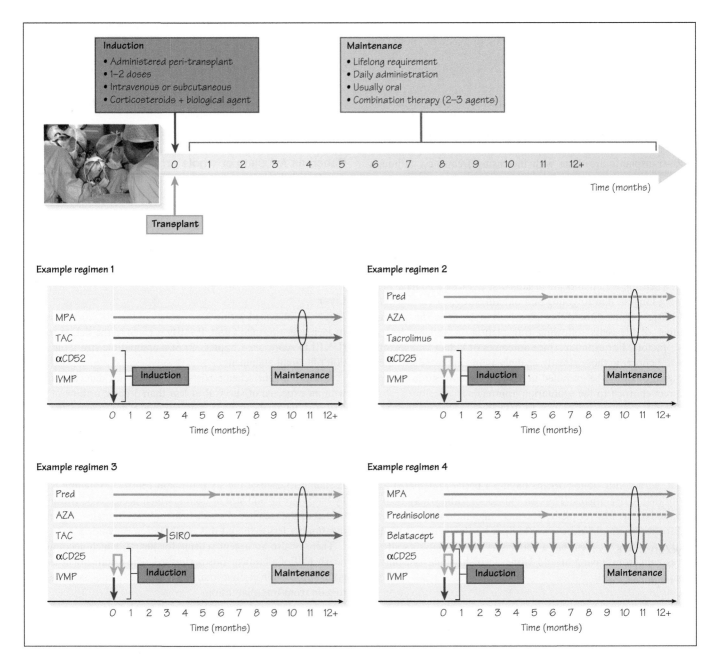

Following organ transplantation, the recipient's immune system identifies the graft as non-self by virtue of differences in donor cell surface markers, such as MHC molecules. An immune response against the graft follows, which will result in the loss of the transplanted organ, unless immunosuppressive agents are used to dampen the immune response.

During the early post-transplant period, patients are at high risk of rejection. Therefore, an intense *induction* regimen of immunosuppressive agents is used, which usually involves the administration of intravenous or subcutaneous agents, often a combination of intravenous corticosteroids together with a biological agent (*see* Chapter 15). Some centres (particularly in North America) use lymphocyte-depleting antibodies such as anti-thymocyte globulin (ATG) or the

monoclonal antibody alemtuzumab (CamPath-1H). In the UK, many centres use an anti-CD25 monoclonal antibody (basiliximab).

Following induction therapy, the patient will require long-term *maintenance* immunosuppression. In contrast to induction agents, these are administered orally, and often consist of triple therapy (for example, a combination of prednisolone (tapering dose), a calcineurin inhibitor such as ciclosporin or tacrolimus, and an anti-proliferative agent such as azathioprine or mycophenolate). If acute rejection does occur, a further intensification of immunosuppression is required, involving the administration of intravenous corticosteroids. The exact immunosuppresive regimen used usually depends on the patient, and balancing their risk of developing rejection with their likely susceptibility to side-effects.

Transplantation at a Glance, First Edition. Menna Clatworthy, Christopher Watson, Michael Allison and John Dark.

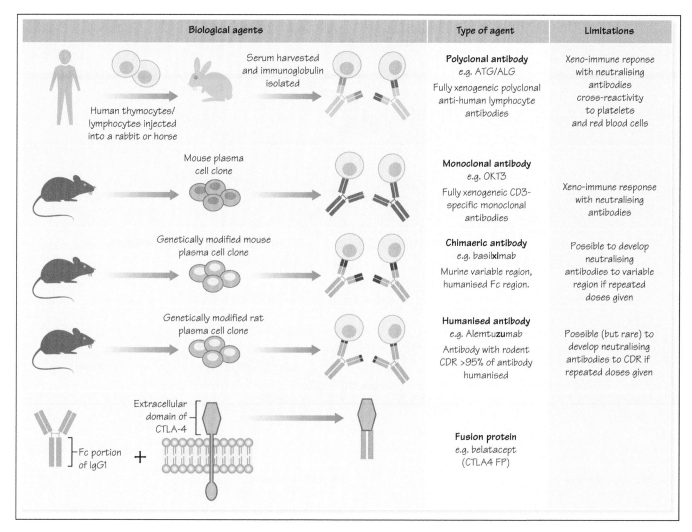

Biological agents	Type of agent	Limitations
Human thymocytes/lymphocytes injected into a rabbit or horse. Serum harvested and immunoglobulin isolated	**Polyclonal antibody** e.g. ATG/ALG. Fully xenogeneic polyclonal anti-human lymphocyte antibodies	Xeno-immune reponse with neutralising antibodies cross-reactivity to platelets and red blood cells
Mouse plasma cell clone	**Monoclonal antibody** e.g. OKT3. Fully xenogeneic CD3-specific monoclonal antibodies	Xeno-immune response with neutralising antibodies
Genetically modified mouse plasma cell clone	**Chimaeric antibody** e.g. basilximab. Murine variable region, humanised Fc region.	Possible to develop neutralising antibodies to variable region if repeated doses given
Genetically modified rat plasma cell clone	**Humanised antibody** e.g. Alemtuzumab. Antibody with rodent CDR >95% of antibody humanised	Possible (but rare) to develop neutralising antibodies to CDR if repeated doses given
Fc portion of IgG1 + Extracellular domain of CTLA-4	**Fusion protein** e.g. belatacept (CTLA4 FP)	

Polyclonal antibodies

Polyclonal antibodies, such as anti-thymocyte globulin (ATG) and anti-lymphocyte globulin (ALG), are prepared by inoculating rabbits or horses with human lymphocytes or thymocytes and collecting their serum following immunisation. The IgG fraction is purified, but contains antibodies not only to lymphocytes, but also to platelets and red cells. ATG and ALG are fully xenogeneic and are therefore recognised by the recipient's immune system as foreign, resulting in the development of neutralising antibodies. This prevents recurrent use. Despite this limitation, the lack of specificity and the development of a first-dose reaction, the so-called 'cytokine release syndrome' that follows cell lysis in up to 80% of patients, ATG is still used to treat steroid-resistant rejection.

Monoclonal antibodies

Monoclonal antibodies (mAbs) are derived from a single plasma cell clone, and thus have a single specificity. The first mAb used in transplantation was the anti-CD3 antibody Muromonab-CD3 (OKT3). This has the advantage of specificity, targeting only T cells, but patients may still develop a cytokine release syndrome. Furthermore, OKT3 is a fully xenogeneic protein and thus anti-bodies are raised against it, limiting efficacy. Newer mAb are comprised of a murine variable region and a human Fc portion (chimeric antibodies, e.g. basiliximab) or are more fully humanised with only a xenogenic complementarity-determining region (CDR), e.g. alemtuzumab, where the CDRs are of rat origin. The nomenclature of mAbs allows the identification of the source of antibody by the letters preceding the mAb stem. For chimeric antibodies, the source substem '-xi-' are used, whereas for humanised antibodies, the substem '-zu-' is used. All mAb now end with the stem-mab.

Fusion proteins

An alternative to humanised mAbs is the construction of fusion proteins (FPs), in which the Fc part of human IgG1 is fused with a human soluble receptor or ligand of a target molecule. FPs are novel molecules but are composed of fully human subunits, limiting the development of neutralising antibodies. The addition of the Fc portion of IgG1 prolongs the half-life of the soluble receptor or ligand. In transplantation, belatacept, a modified CTLA-4 fusion protein, has been used as a maintenance agent in place of calcineurin inhibitors.

Transplantation at a Glance, First Edition. Menna Clatworthy, Christopher Watson, Michael Allison and John Dark.

16 T cell-targeted immunosuppression

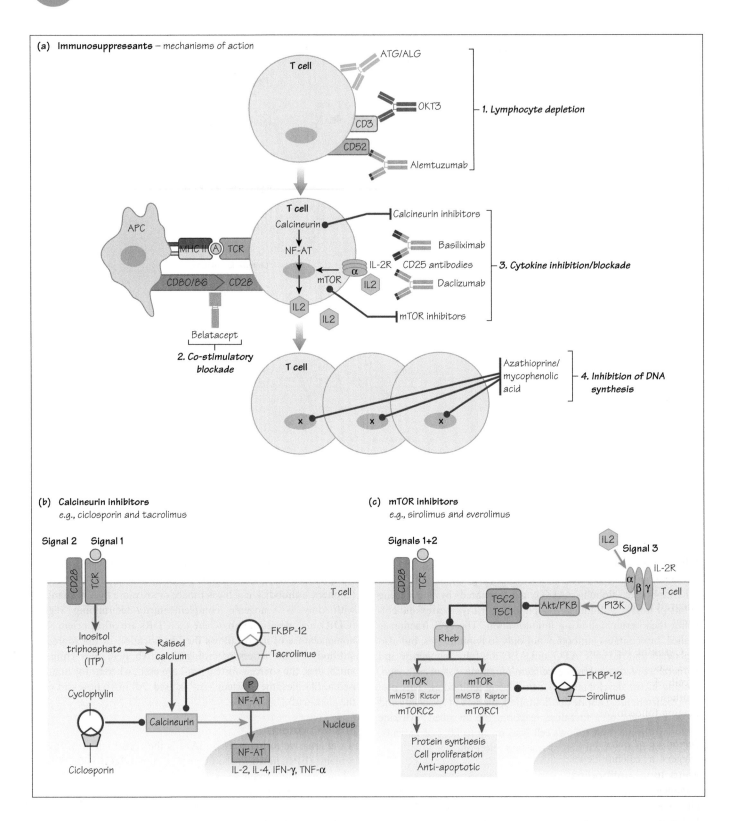

The most common form of rejection encountered is T cell-mediated (TMR) (also known as acute cellular rejection (ACR)), occurring in 15–20% of transplants. ACR is characterised histologically by lymphocyte infiltration into the graft (predominantly cytotoxic [CD8] T cells). ACR is orchestrated by CD4 T cells, which are activated by antigen-presenting cells (APCs), such as dendritic cells and B cells, presenting donor antigen to CD4 T cells via MHC class II molecules. For full activation of T cells, APCs also provide a co-stimulatory signal via surface molecules such as CD80/86. Such activated T cells produce large quantities of cytokines, particularly interleukin (IL)-2, which further drive the activation and proliferation of both CD4 and CD8 T cells. Thus, immunosuppressive agents predominantly target T cell activation via four broad mechanisms.

1. Lymphocyte depletion

Lymphocyte depletion has been achieved using biological agents (*see* Chapter 15), initially polyclonal agents such as ATG and ALG or the T cell-specific anti-CD3 antibody OKT3. Alemtuzumab (CamPath-1H) is a humanised rat IgG1 monoclonal antibody that binds CD52, a glycoprotein present on the surface of lymphocytes, dendritic cells and natural killer (NK) cells. Administration of alemtuzumab leads to rapid and sustained depletion of both T and B lymphocytes. It is principally used at induction and allows a corticosteroid-free maintenance regimen.

2. Disruption of T cell activation by co-stimulatory blockade

When T cells are activated by APCs two signals are required for full activation. First, the T cell receptor must recognise and bind to its specific antigen presented in the context of MHC. The second signal is mediated by the engagement of pairs of co-stimulatory molecules expressed on the surface of T cells and APCs, for example CD28 (T cell) and B7 (also known as CD80/CD86, found on APCs).

CTLA4 is a molecule present on the surface of T cells and is a competitive inhibitor of the CD28:B7 interaction. CTLA4-Ig (abatacept) consists of the extracellular domain of human CTLA4 linked to the Fc portion of IgG1. Abatacept blocks co-stimulation via the CD28:B7 pathway, and in rodent models has prevented rejection of cardiac, renal, pancreatic, hepatic and skin allografts. However, in non-human primate models, abatacept is an ineffective means of prophylaxis against rejection. This led to the modification of abatacept to produce more avid binding to CD86 and thus more potent inhibition of T cell activation. The result was belatacept (LEA29Y), a fusion protein that differed from abatacept by two amino acids. Belatacept is effective in preventing allograft rejection in humans and has been used as a maintenance agent.

3. Cytokine blockade

IL-2 acts as a potent activator and pro-proliferative cytokine for T cells. A number of agents have been developed that inhibit IL-2 synthesis, IL-2 binding to its cell surface receptor, or signal transduction following IL-2 receptor ligation.

Inhibition of cytokine synthesis Antigen presentation to T cells triggers a calcium-dependent intracellular signalling cascade, which results in the activation of the phosphatase calcineurin. Calcineurin dephosphorylates the transcription factor NF-AT, allowing its translocation to the nucleus, where it enhances the transcription of a number of cytokines, including IL-2. Calcineurin inhibitors (CNIs) such as ciclosporin and tacrolimus form complexes with intracellular immunophilins (cyclophilin and FK506-binding protein respectively). These CNI–immunophilin complexes

inhibit calcineurin and thus prevent the translocation of NF-AT to the nucleus and inhibit its subsequent actions there. CNIs are useful maintenance immunosuppressants but are nephrotoxic, leading to chronic graft dysfunction.

Corticosteroids, for example prednisolone, have a variety of anti-inflammatory effects including suppression of prostaglandin synthesis, reduction of histamine and bradykinin release, and the inhibition of the production of several pro-inflammatory cytokines. They are widely used and still form a part of many maintenance regimens. In addition, they are also used as first-line treatment of ACR.

Inhibition of IL-2 receptor binding The effects of IL-2 on T cells are dependent on binding to its cell surface receptor. The IL-2 receptor has three subunits, α (CD25), β and γ. During T cell activation the α subunit becomes associated with the other subunits to form a high-affinity receptor. Blockade of the IL-2 receptor by targeting the α-chain profoundly inhibits T cell proliferation. One anti-CD25mAb, basiliximab, is currently in wide clinical use as an induction agent in renal transplantation. Another, daclizumab, has been recently withdrawn from use. Both have proven efficacy in the reduction of the incidence and severity of ACR in renal transplantation.

Inhibition of signal transduction Sirolimus (rapamycin) and everolimus bind to the FK506 binding protein and the resulting complex inhibits an intracellular kinase, the mammalian target of rapamycin complex 1 (mTORC1). mTORC1 is important in a variety of signalling pathways, including that found downstream of the IL-2 receptor. Thus, inhibition of mTORC1 blocks both T cell activation and proliferation by preventing cell-cycle progression. In addition, sirolimus and everolimus also inhibit the VEGF pathway and thus have anti-angiogenic effects, a property that has been used for the treatment of some cancers (e.g. Kaposi's sarcoma).

4. Inhibition of DNA synthesis

For lymphocytes to proliferate, they must synthesise new DNA prior to division. Thus, agents that inhibit DNA synthesis act as useful immunosuppressants.

Azathioprine (AZA) is a pro-drug which is converted into the purine analogue 6-mercaptopurine (6-MP). It was first used in the early 1960s in renal transplantation and continues to be used in many centres as part of a maintenance regimen. The main disadvantage of azathioprine is that of non-specific bone marrow suppression. The enzyme thiopurine S-methyltransferase (TPMT) deactivates 6-MP, and genetic polymorphisms of TPMT, which are associated with loss of function, can lead to drug toxicity.

Mycophenolate mofetil (MMF) and mycophenolate sodium (MPS) are also pro-drugs, converted in the liver to mycophenolic acid (MPA). MPA is a non-competitive, reversible inhibitor of inosine monophosphate dehydrogenase (IMPDH), the enzyme that controls the rate of synthesis of guanine monophosphate in the *de novo* pathway of purine synthesis. Most cells can generate guanosine nucleotides by two pathways, the IMPDH pathway and the salvage pathway. Lymphocytes lack this salvage pathway, thus MPA specifically targets lymphocytes while sparing other cells. MPA now forms part of the maintenance immunosuppressive protocol of many transplant centres.

	SRL	CIC	Tac	MPA	Aza	Pred
Nephrotoxicity	–	++	++	–	–	–
Hypertension	–	+	+	–	–	+
Dyslipidaemia	+++	++	+	–	–	+
Diabetogenic	–	+	+++	–	–	++
Hyperuricaemia	–	+	+	–	–	–
Neurotoxicity	–	++	++	–	–	+
Anaemia	+	–	–	+	+	–
Leucopenia	+	–	–	+	+	–
Platelets	+	–	–	+	+	–
Skin and gums	+	++	–	–	–	+
Osteoporosis	–	+	+	–	–	++
GI upset	+	–	–	++	–	–

Corticosteroids (Cushingoid features)

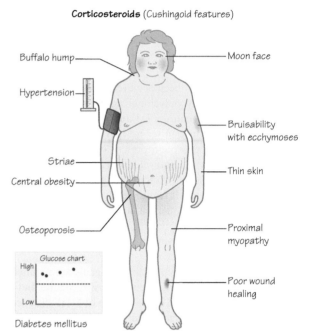

- Buffalo hump
- Hypertension
- Striae
- Central obesity
- Osteoporosis
- Moon face
- Bruisability with ecchymoses
- Thin skin
- Proximal myopathy
- Poor wound healing

Glucose chart — High / Low

Diabetes mellitus

Calcineurin inhibitors

Ciclosporin

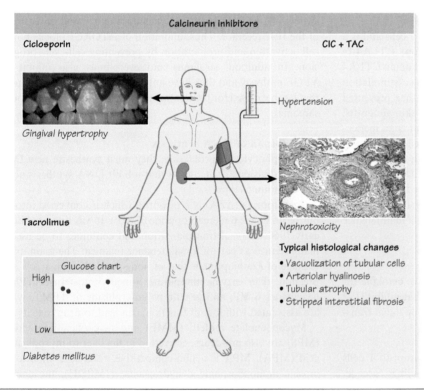

Gingival hypertrophy

Tacrolimus

Glucose chart — High / Low

Diabetes mellitus

CIC + TAC

Hypertension

Nephrotoxicity

Typical histological changes
- Vacuolization of tubular cells
- Arteriolar hyalinosis
- Tubular atrophy
- Stripped interstitial fibrosis

Anti-proliferative agents

MPA

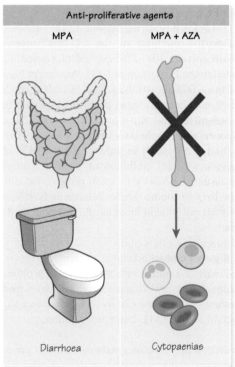

Diarrhoea

MPA + AZA

Cytopaenias

Transplantation at a Glance, First Edition. Menna Clatworthy, Christopher Watson, Michael Allison and John Dark.

40 © 2012 John Wiley & Sons, Ltd. Published 2012 by John Wiley & Sons, Ltd.

Immunosuppressants are necessary to prevent allograft rejection, but these agents have a number of unwanted side effects. These include generic side effects associated with all immunosuppressive agents, such an increased susceptibility to infection and malignancy, and drug-specific side effects.

Corticosteroids

High-dose, intravenous corticosteroids (usually methyl prednisolone) are used at induction and to treat acute cellular rejection. Oral corticosteroids, typically prednisolone, are used for maintenance therapy. Prolonged exposure to corticosteroids results in a number of side effects:
- thinning of the skin and easy bruising
- weight gain with central adiposity and abdominal striae
- proximal myopathy
- osteoporosis
- avascular necrosis
- glucose intolerance/new onset diabetes mellitus
- hypertension
- peptic ulceration.

These adverse effects may be minimised by rapidly tapering steroid dose post-transplant and by using gastric (an H2 blocker or a proton pump inhibitor) and bone protection (vitamin D3 or calcium) in high-risk individuals. Some transplant centres avoid using maintenance corticosteroids because of these side effects.

Calcineurin inhibitors (CNIs)

Although CNIs significantly reduce the risk of acute rejection, and thus revolutionised early graft survival, it was rapidly appreciated that these agents were nephrotoxic. Serial renal biopsies show that CNI toxicity may affect the graft within weeks of transplantation. Typical acute changes include vacuolation of tubular cells. Following chronic exposure there is intimal thickening of arterioles, tubular atrophy and interstitial fibrosis. CNIs are also associated with tremor, which is dose-dependent, and at very high levels or in susceptible patients, may cause fitting.

Specific side effects associated with ciclosporin include hirsuitism and gingival hypertrophy. Tacrolimus is associated with glucose intolerance and a three times increased risk of developing new onset diabetes after transplant (NODAT) compared with ciclosporin.

Anti-metabolites

Azathioprine inhibits purine production and hence DNA synthesis, thus preventing cell division. Associated side effects include bone marrow suppression, resulting in pancytopaenia or isolated leukopaenias. The risk of marrow suppression is increased if high doses are used or if patients have a low-activity polymorphism in the enzyme that breaks down azathioprine (thiopurine methyltransferase [TPMT]).

Mycophenolate specifically inhibits inosine monophosphate dehydrogenase (IMPDH), which is the rate-limiting enzyme in guanine nucleotide synthesis. Its effects are said to be lymphocyte-specific (given that other cells have an alternative salvage pathway for nucleotide synthesis). However, pancytopaenia is frequently observed particularly if prescribed in combination with ganciclovir. Gastrointestinal upset, particularly diarrhoea, is also a common problem.

mTOR inhibitors

The effects of mTOR inhibitors (sirolimus and everolimus) are not limited to immune cells, as mTORC1 is a critical signalling complex in most cells. Associated side effects include dyslipidaemia, skin rashes, mouth ulceration, inhibition of wound healing and an increased risk of lymphocoeles. Interstitial pneumonitis is an uncommon but serious side effect of sirolimus, occurring in around 1% of patients, and requires immediate cessation of the drug. Sirolimus can exacerbate CNI-mediated nephrotoxicity and may cause proteinuria.

Biological agents

Biological agents are usually administered via the intravenous route, and agents that cause cytolysis (e.g. ATG, alemtuzumab) are associated with first-dose reactions (also known as cytokine release syndrome) of varying severity, which may be reduced by pre-medicating with intravenous corticosteroids and an antihistamine, such as chlorpheniramine.

These agents are variably xenogeneic and may incite an immune response, characterised by the development of neutralising antibodies. This may prevent recurrent use and even predispose to anaphylactic reactions during re-challenge.

Polyclonal antibodies

Lymphocyte-depleting agents such as ATG lead to profound immunosuppression and their use has been associated with an increased risk of cytomegalovirus (CMV) infection and post-transplant lymphoproliferative disease (PTLD).

Monoclonal antibodies

The anti-CD25 agents basiliximab and daclizumab are not T cell depleting, and therefore appear to have a very good safety profile.

The anti-CD52 agent alemtuzumab causes lymphocyte depletion but does not appear to be associated with an increased risk of CMV infection. Its use has been linked with the subsequent development of antibody-mediated autoimmune diseases, for example, immune thrombocytopaenia and haemolytic anaemia.

18 Post-transplant infection

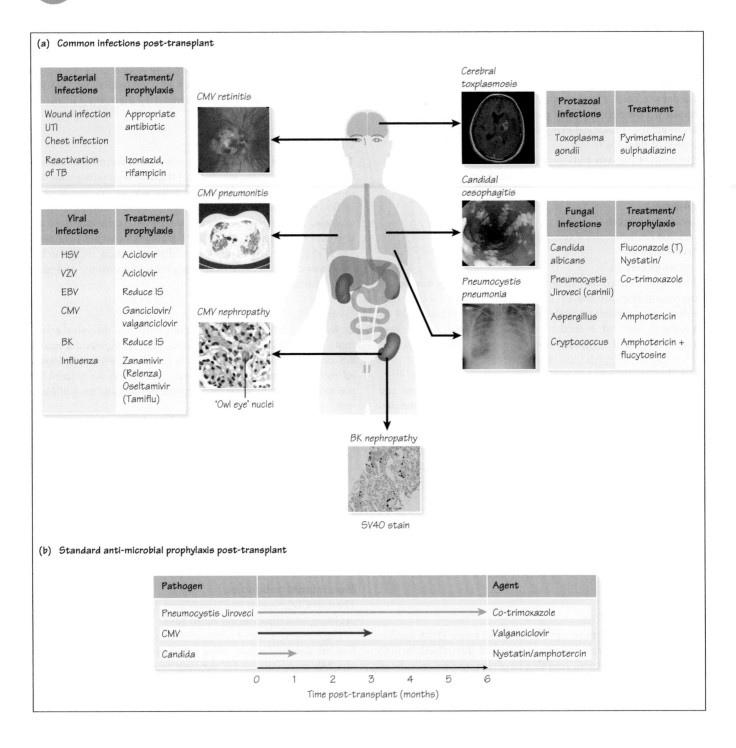

(a) Common infections post-transplant

Bacterial infections	Treatment/ prophylaxis
Wound infection UTI Chest infection	Appropriate antibiotic
Reactivation of TB	Izoniazid, rifampicin

Viral infections	Treatment/ prophylaxis
HSV	Aciclovir
VZV	Aciclovir
EBV	Reduce IS
CMV	Ganciclovir/ valganciclovir
BK	Reduce IS
Influenza	Zanamivir (Relenza) Oseltamivir (Tamiflu)

CMV retinitis

CMV pneumonitis

CMV nephropathy

'Owl eye' nuclei

Cerebral toxoplasmosis

Protazoal infections	Treatment
Toxoplasma gondii	Pyrimethamine/ sulphadiazine

Candidal oesophagitis

Pneumocystis pneumonia

Fungal infections	Treatment/ prophylaxis
Candida albicans	Fluconazole (T) Nystatin/
Pneumocystis Jiroveci (carinii)	Co-trimoxazole
Aspergillus	Amphotericin
Cryptococcus	Amphotericin + flucytosine

BK nephropathy

SV40 stain

(b) Standard anti-microbial prophylaxis post-transplant

Pathogen		Agent
Pneumocystis Jiroveci		Co-trimoxazole
CMV		Valganciclovir
Candida		Nystatin/amphotercin

Time post-transplant (months)
0 1 2 3 4 5 6

Following transplantation, patients are given immunosuppressive agents to prevent rejection. Unfortunately, this inevitably increases susceptibility to infection. Post-transplant immunosuppression has significant effects on T lymphocytes, hence many of the opportunistic infections seen are similar to those observed in patients with HIV, particularly cytomegalovirus (CMV) and *Pneumocystis jiroveci (*previously called *P. carinii*). In the early post-transplant period (months 1–3), immunosuppression is relatively intense, and therefore the patient is at particular risk of more unusual, opportunistic infection. In addition, some immunosuppressive agents are more powerful than others, e.g. lymphocyte-depleting agents such as ATG. Use of ATG at induction carries a higher risk of subsequent infection than the use of non-depleting biological agents such as anti-CD25 monoclonal antibodies. When considering infections occurring post-transplant, they can be divided according to causative agents.

Transplantation at a Glance, First Edition. Menna Clatworthy, Christopher Watson, Michael Allison and John Dark.

Viral infections

Transplant immunosuppression is associated with reactivation of a number of latent viral infections including cytomegalovirus (CMV), varicella zoster virus (VZV), herpes simplex virus (HSV), Epstein-Barr virus (EBV) and BK virus, and also increases the severity of disease during primary infection with these viruses such that they may be life threatening.

1 CMV – CMV is a γ-herpes virus and is one of the most common infections encountered post-transplant. CMV infection can present with non-specific symptoms such as fever, sweats, lethargy and weight loss. CMV can affect specific organs such as the gut (CMV colitis), the eyes (CMV retinitis, 'brush fire' appearance), the lungs (CMV pneumonitis), the liver and the allograft (*see* Chapter 19).

2 VZV – between 80 and 90% of adults have a previous history of chicken pox. Thereafter the virus lies dormant in dorsal root ganglia and may subsequently reactivate post-transplant, presenting with a vesicular, painful rash in a dermatomal distribution (shingles).

3 HSV1/2 – between 80 and 90% of adults have latent HSV1 infection which can reactivate post-transplant, presenting as oral ulceration ('cold sores'). HSV1 can also cause gastrointestinal (GI) disease and encephalitis in the immunocompromised. HSV2 infection is less common and presents with genital ulceration. Treatment is with aciclovir.

4 EBV – more than 90% of adults have evidence of previous EBV infection (seropositive for EBV-specific IgG). The virus subsequently establishes latent infection in B cells. Primary EBV infection (infectious mononucleosis) post-transplant can be extremely severe and may be associated with the development of lymphoma (*see* Chapter 20).

5 BK virus – BK virus is a double-stranded DNA virus of the *Polyomaviridae* family. Approximately 70–90% of the adult population have evidence of previous infection. Primary infection is usually asymptomatic, but the virus establishes latency within the genitourinary tract. Reactivation is common in renal transplant recipients (viraemia is detectable in 10–20% of patients in the first year post-transplant). Around half of these will have biopsy-proven BK nephropathy (i.e. 5–10% transplant recipients). Patients with BK nephropathy are asymptomatic and present with a decline in allograft function. Renal transplant biopsy is required for diagnosis. Typical biopsy changes include interstitial inflammation, which can progress to interstitial fibrosis and tubular atrophy. The biopsy should be stained with an SV40 antibody, which stains BK virus within tubular cells. BK infection has also been associated with the development of ureteric stenosis. The main risk factor for the development of BK nephropathy is the use of more intense immunosuppressive regimens.

BK virus can be detected by performing polymerase chain reaction (PCR) on blood or urine samples or by cytopathological examination of urine for the presence of decoy cells (uroepithelial cells with nuclear inclusions). There is no specific antiviral therapy for BK virus. The main strategy is to decrease immunosuppression. Ciprofloxacin, leflunomide, cidofovir and IVIg have all been used to treat BK nephropathy, but there is no randomised control trial data to support their use.

Fungal infections

1 *Candida albicans* is a commensal organism which is found on the skin, and in the genital and GI tracts. Immunosuppression is associated with the development of symptomatic infection, including oropharyngeal candidiasis ('thrush') and candidal oesophagitis. Candidal species may also cause infections of intravascular and peritoneal dialysis catheters. Rarely, patients can develop invasive disease and fungaemia. Other candidal species observed post-transplant include *C. glabrata*, which is resistant to fluconazole and therefore difficult to treat. Patients are usually given prophylaxis in the first 4–6 weeks post transplant (oral nystatin). Treatment for symptomatic infection is oral fluconazole and for invasive disease intravenous amphotericin B or caspofungin.

2 *Pneumocystis jiroveci* (**previously *P. carinii***) is a ubiquitous environmental fungus that causes symptomatic infection in a third of transplant recipients in the absence of prophylaxis. Patients present with a dry cough and shortness of breath and may have normal oxygen saturations at rest, but become rapidly hypoxic on exertion. At presentation, chest signs and chest X-ray (CXR) changes are often scant, relative to the degree hypoxia observed. Diagnosis is usually made by examination of bronchoalveolar lavage (BAL) fluid or transbronchial biopsy. Treatment is with co-trimoxazole. Most transplant centres also offer prophylaxis in the first 6 months post transplant.

3 *Aspergillus fumigatus* is the most commonly observed aspergillus species in transplant recipients. It is acquired from the environment by inhalation of spores. It frequently causes lung disease (often cavitating lesions on CXR), forming nodules, which can be invasive and erode into blood vessels. It may also become disseminated infecting heart, kidneys and brain, portending an extremely poor prognosis. Diagnosis is usually by examination of BAL, which demonstrates fungal hyphae. Treatment is with IV amphotericin B, voriconazole or caspofungin.

4 *Cryptococcus neoformans* can cause pulmonary disease (nodules, pneumonia) and meningitis. Diagnosis is by India ink staining of cerebrospinal fluid (CSF) or by serology. Treatment is with IV amphotericin B and flucytosine.

Protozoal infections

Toxoplasma gondii is the most commonly observed protozoal infection post-transplant. Infection occurs via ingestion of meat contaminated with cysts. It causes cerebral lesions and encephalitis. Treatment is with pyrimethamine and sulphadiazine.

Bacterial infections

Most early infections are related to the transplant procedure and include infections of the wound (usually caused by staphylococci), urinary tract infections (*Escherichia coli*) and chest infections (pneumococci or atypical organisms). In addition, haemodialysis catheters or peritoneal dialysis catheters may also become infected peri-operatively.

Later problems include chest infections, sinusitis, dental abscess and endocarditis, which may be caused by more unusual organisms, e.g. nocardia, listeria. Healthcare-associated infections (HAI), for example methicillin-resistant *Staphylococcus aureus* (MRSA), *Clostridium difficile* and vancomycin-resistant enterococci (VRE), may also be a problem in patients who require recurrent hospital admissions for post-transplant complications.

Latent *Mycobacterium tuberculosis* infection may be reactivated by immunosuppression. Individuals at risk of reactivation or primary mycobacterial infection should be placed on prophylaxis at the time of transplantation.

19 CMV infection

(a) Primary infection in immunocompetant

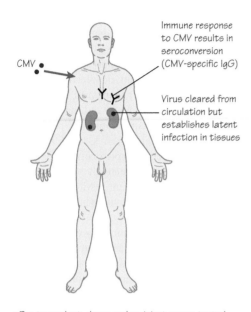

Immune response to CMV results in seroconversion (CMV-specific IgG)

CMV

Virus cleared from circulation but establishes latent infection in tissues

- Pre-transplant, donor and recipient serum tested
- Donor serum:
  - CMV IgG absent = **D−**
  - CMV IgG present = **D+**
- Recipient serum:
  - CMV IgG absent = **R−**
  - CMV IgG present = **R+**

(b) CMV in transplantation

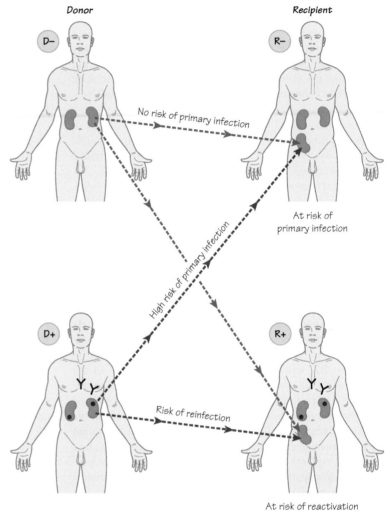

Donor

Recipient

D−

R−

No risk of primary infection

At risk of primary infection

High risk of primary infection

D+

R+

Risk of reinfection

At risk of reactivation or reinfection

(c) CMV resistance to ganciclovir

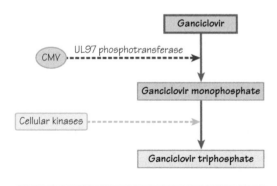

Ganciclovir

CMV — UL97 phosphotransferase →

Ganciclovir monophosphate

Cellular kinases

Ganciclovir triphosphate

Mutations in CMV gene encoding UL97 PT render ganciclovir ineffective, as this enzyme is required to convert the drug to its active form

(d) Risk of CMV infection post transplant

CMV mismatch	Viraemia	CMV disease*
D−R−	0	0
D−R+	25%	15%
D+R+	55%	25%
D+R−	75%	60%

* CMV disease = symptomatic infection

Transplantation at a Glance, First Edition. Menna Clatworthy, Christopher Watson, Michael Allison and John Dark.

Risk of CMV infection post transplant

Cytomegalovirus (CMV) is a γ-herpes virus and is one of the most common infections encountered post-transplant. The likelihood of infection post-transplant is dependent on whether the recipient has had previous CMV infection and therefore has immunological memory of the virus. Immune memory is detected by looking for the presence of CMV-specific antibody (IgG).

Around 50% of adults in the UK are CMV immune (seropositive) and 50% seronegative. Seronegative transplant recipients (R–) who receive an allograft from a CMV seropositive donor (D+) are at risk of developing primary infection; in the absence of prophylaxis, 60% will develop symptomatic CMV infection post transplant. Thus, most transplant centres would give CMV prophylaxis to this high-risk group of recipients in the form of oral valganciclovir. Many centres also offer 'universal prophylaxis' to all at risk patients (D+R–, D–R+, D+R+).

Clinical features of CMV infection

The presentation of post-transplant CMV is very variable; infection can be relatively asymptomatic in patients with immunological memory to the virus and is diagnosed only by routine screening by polymerase chain reaction (PCR). In others, particularly those who develop primary infection while immunosuppressed, it can be life-threatening. Systemic symptoms associated with CMV include fever, sweats, lethargy and weight loss. Abdominal pain may accompany gastrointestinal (GI) infection or pancreatitis. CMV can also present with organ-specific disease, including:
• colitis – symptoms include diarrhoea and weight loss
• retinitis – typical retinal appearance is of a 'brush fire'
• pneumonitis – patients present with breathlessness, widespread alveolar infiltrates visible on chest radiograph or CT
• allograft – viral inclusions can be observed on renal transplant biopsy, and are usually associated with a decline in allograft function, even in the absence of rejection.

Diagnosis

CMV is diagnosed by the detection of virus particles in the blood (viraemia) or in urine. PCR performed on blood/urine samples allows the identification of viral DNA. Alternatively, classical 'owl eye' inclusion bodies may be observed within the nuclei of infected cells isolated by biopsy or bronchio-alveolar lavage by histology or cytology. CMV-specific antibodies can also be used in immunohistochemical staining of biopsy material.

Treatment

CMV should be treated in the following ways.
• *Reduction in immunosuppression* – the development of a CMV infection suggests that the patient is relatively over-immunosuppressed. Usually the target trough level of calcineurin inhibitor (CNI) is reduced and the antiproliferative agent (azathioprine or mycophenolate) stopped.
• *Specific treatment for CMV* – intravenous ganciclovir is the treatment of choice for patients with life-threatening disease. Patients with low viral titres or with reactivation rather than primary disease can be treated with high-dose oral valganciclovir. Valganciclovir is a pro-drug which is converted in the liver to ganciclovir. Ganciclovir must be phosphorylated in order to generate its active metabolite ganciclovir triphosphate. Phosphorylation is dependent in part on a CMV-synthesised enzyme UL97 phosphotransferase. Thus, the virus may become resistant to ganciclovir if it mutates to produce a non-functional enzyme.
• Other agents used include foscarnet, cidofovir and intravenous CMV immune globulin, although these are usually reserved for patients with refractory or ganciclovir resistant disease.

Complications of CMV infection

Studies suggest that CMV infection (either symptomatic or asymptomatic) can have an adverse effect on both patient and allograft survival. CMV infection has been associated with:
• acute rejection
• chronic allograft nephropathy (CMV infection induces fibrosis and vascular thickening in animal models of transplantation). Such chronic changes together with an increase in acute rejection reduce long-term allograft survival
• cardiovascular complications, thus a reduced patient survival
• post-transplant diabetes mellitus.

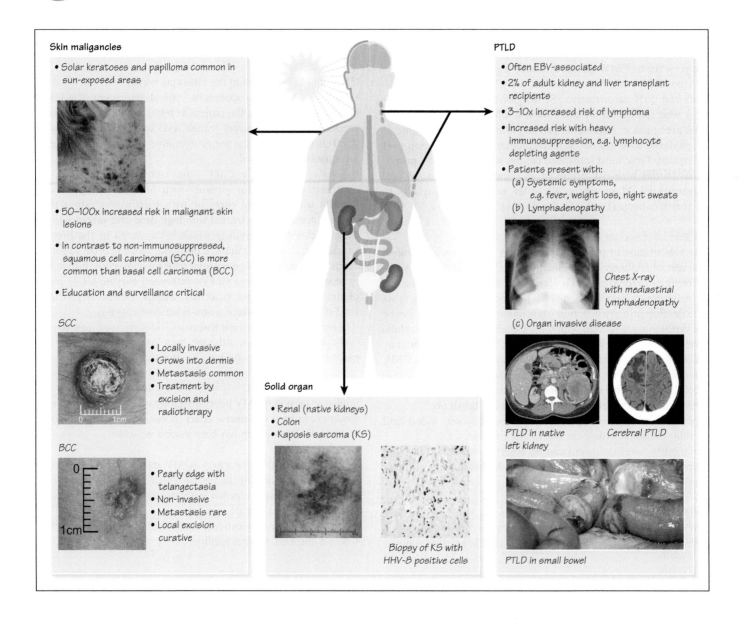

Skin maligancies

- Solar keratoses and papilloma common in sun-exposed areas

- 50–100x increased risk in malignant skin lesions

- In contrast to non-immunosuppressed, squamous cell carcinoma (SCC) is more common than basal cell carcinoma (BCC)

- Education and surveillance critical

SCC

- Locally invasive
- Grows into dermis
- Metastasis common
- Treatment by excision and radiotherapy

BCC

- Pearly edge with telangectasia
- Non-invasive
- Metastasis rare
- Local excision curative

Solid organ

- Renal (native kidneys)
- Colon
- Kaposis sarcoma (KS)

Biopsy of KS with HHV-8 positive cells

PTLD

- Often EBV-associated
- 2% of adult kidney and liver transplant recipients
- 3–10x increased risk of lymphoma
- Increased risk with heavy immunosuppression, e.g. lymphocyte depleting agents
- Patients present with:
  (a) Systemic symptoms, e.g. fever, weight loss, night sweats
  (b) Lymphadenopathy

Chest X-ray with mediastinal lymphadenopathy

(c) Organ invasive disease

PTLD in native left kidney

Cerebral PTLD

PTLD in small bowel

The use of immunosuppressive therapy has led to a significant reduction in rejection, and a consequent improvement in graft and patient survival. Thus, many transplant recipients will be exposed to immunosuppressants for years or even decades. One of the major complications of prolonged immunosuppression is an increased risk of malignancy, particularly those driven by oncoviruses such as human papilloma virus (HPV) and Epstein-Barr virus (EBV). In addition, immunosuppressive drugs inhibit immune tumour surveillance, potentiate the effects of other carcinogens such as ultraviolet (UV) light, and some agents directly promote tumour formation or progression (for example ciclosporin stimulates vascular endothelial growth factor [VEGF]-A-associated tumour vascularisation and increases TGF-β production).

Incidence of malignancy

Overall, the frequency of malignancy is at least twofold higher in transplant recipients compared with the normal population. Skin malignancies are 15–200 times more common (depending on sun exposure). The incidence of solid organ malignancies is also increased; roughly speaking, a transplant recipient's risk of developing a malignancy is similar to a normal individual 10–20 years older than them.

Risk factors

1 *Exposure to UV light* – patients with high exposure to UV light (e.g. those in sunny climates such as in Australia) have a 100- to 200-fold increased risk of non-melanotic skin cancers, compared with a 20 times increased risk in those in less sun-exposed environments such as the UK.

2 *Previous exposure to immunosuppressants* as treatments for primary disease, e.g. cyclophosphamide treatment for vasculitis or lupus nephritis increases the risk of bladder cancer and of lymphoproliferative diseases.

3 *Long-term uraemia* – patients with end-stage renal failure (ESRF) on dialysis have an increased risk of malignancy, perhaps due to an accumulation of carcinogenic toxins.

4 *Chronic viral infection* – both hepatitis B and hepatitis C infection increase the risk of hepatocellular carcinoma.

Types of cancer
Post-transplant lymphoproliferative disease (PTLD)

PTLD is the most common type of cancer observed in paediatric transplant recipients, and the second most common in adults, occurring in 2% of adult kidney and liver transplant recipients. Patients exposed to heavy immunosuppression, particularly lymphocyte-depleting agents such as ATG, are at increased risk of PTLD. Most PTLD is driven by EBV; primary EBV infection in immunocompetent individuals results in infectious mononucleosis. The virus subsequently establishes latency in B lymphocytes. When primary infection occurs in a transplant recipient receiving immunosuppression, e.g. an EBV-naive recipient receiving a transplant from an EBV-positive donor, the individual may develop a more severe mononucleosis-like illness and in some cases an aggressive lymphoma. Children are more likely to be EBV-naive, hence the increased incidence of PTLD in this population. Fifty per cent of cases of PTLD are diagnosed within the first two years post-transplant. Presenting features include local effects (e.g. fitting in cerebral PTLD, abdominal pain if gastrointestinal involvement, local swelling secondary to lymphadenopathy, and transplant dysfunction if there is graft infiltration). Systemic symptoms include fever, night sweats, and weight loss. The diagnosis is confirmed by tissue biopsy, which allows its classification into three categories.

1 Diffuse B cell hyperplasia: EBV-positive, normal lymphoid architecture.

2 Polymorphic PTLD: usually EBV-positive, polymorphic atypical lymphocytes disrupting lymphoid architechture.

3 Monomorphic PTLD: often EBV-negative; high-grade malignant B or T cell lymphoma.

Treatment is dependent on type/severity of disease and includes:

• Reduction in immunosuppression to allow the patient to mount an immune response to EBV.

• Rituximab, a chimeric anti-CD20 monoclonal antibody which causes depletion of CD20-positive cells. CD20 is expressed by most B cells, thus rituximab is effective in B cell lymphomas.

• Systemic chemotherapy is reserved for patients with monomorphic PTLD.

• Radiotherapy.

• Surgery.

Skin cancers

Non-melanoma skin cancers are the most commonly observed post-transplant malignancy in adults. The main risk factors are UV exposure, fair skin, HPV and prolonged duration of immunosuppression. Thus, 50–75% of Caucasian transplant recipients will be affected by skin malignancies 20 years post transplant. Given the importance of sun exposure, transplant recipients are advised to apply high factor sun blocking cream and to wear protective clothing (e.g. hat, long-sleeved shirt) when in the sun.

Both squamous cell carcinomas (SCC) and basal cell carcinomas (BCC) are observed post-transplant, with SCCs three times more common than BCCs (in contrast to skin cancers in the normal population, where BCCs predominate). SCCs also commonly develop on the lip (60-fold more common than normal population), anus (10-fold) and perineum, all in part driven by HPV.

The good thing about skin cancers is that screening is relatively easy, and most transplant centres routinely perform regular skin surveillance in long-term transplant recipients and encourage patients to perform their own screening.

Treatment of skin malignancies is by local excision and topical cytotoxic agents (e.g. 5-fluorouracil). The use of sirolimus rather than calcineurin inhibitors as maintenance immunosuppression seems to lower the risk of skin cancer, therefore a switch to sirolimus following diagnosis may be beneficial.

Malignant melanomas are also more common in transplant recipients, although the increased risk is much less than for SCCs and BCCs (threefold more common than normal population).

Transplant recipients are also at increased risk of Kaposi's sarcoma (KS), for which human herpes virus (HHV)-8 is the principal aetiological agent. Sirolimus may be useful in reducing VEGFA-mediated stimulation of this endothelial-derived malignancy.

Transplant-specific solid organ cancers

Kidney transplant recipients have an eightfold increased risk of kidney cancer, and a threefold increased risk of multiple myeloma.

Liver transplant recipients have a tenfold increased incidence of oral cancer and higher risk of oesophageal cancer, possibly reflecting lifestyle risks associated with alcohol ingestion, such as cigarette smoking. Treatment is as for the general population, as well as a reduction in immunosuppression where possible.

(a) Temporal classification of renal failure

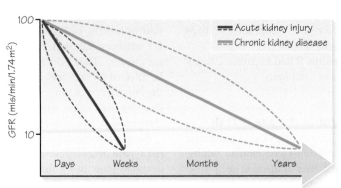

	Acute kidney injury (AKI)	Chronic kidney disease (CKD)
Onset	Days – weeks	Months – years
Aetiology	Pre-renal > Post-renal > Renal	Renal > Post-renal > Pre-renal

(b) Aetiological classification of renal failure

Pre-renal
- Hypotension, sepsis
- Renovascular disease

Post-renal
- Prostatic hypertrophy/cancer
- Bladder pathology (stones, cancer)
- Vesicourteric reflux

Renal
- Glomerular pathology
  - Glomerulonephritis (1°, 2° to lupus, vasculitis), diabetic nephropathy
- Interstitial pathology
  - Interstitial nephritis, chronic pyelonephritis
- Vascular pathology
  - Thrombic microangiopathy, hypertensive nephropathy
- Tubular pathology
  - Acute tubular necrosis, cast nephropathy

(c) Staging of AKI and CKD

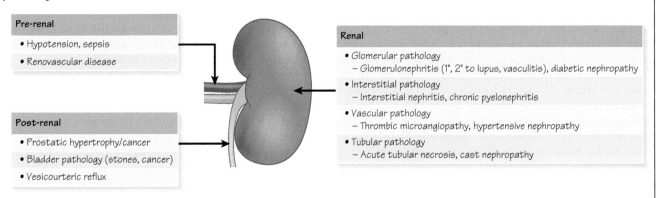

AKI stage	Serum creatinine	Urine output criteria
1	Increase of >26.4 µmol/L (0.3 mg/dL) **or** 150–200% of baseline (1.5–2 increase)	<0.5 ml/kg/hour >6 hours
2	Increase to >200–300% of baseline (2–3 fold increase)	<0.5 ml/kg/hour >12 hours
3	>354 µmol/L (4 mg/dL) with an acute rise of at least 44 µmol/L (0.5 mg/dL) **or** >300% of baseline (3 fold increase)	<0.3 ml/kg/hour >24 hours or anuria for 12 hours

CKD stage	eGFR (ml/min/1.73 m²)	Other features
1	90+	Normal renal function but urine dipstick abnormalities or known structural abnormality of renal tract or diagnosis of genetic kidney disease
2	60–89	Mildly reduced renal function plus urine/structural abnormalities or diagnosis of genetic kidney disease
3	30–59	Moderately reduced renal function
4	15–29	Severely reduced renal function
5	<15	End-stage renal failure

Classification of renal failure

End-stage renal failure (ESRF), as evidenced by a decline in glomerular filtration rate (GFR) such that function is inadequate for health, is relatively common and the prevalence increases with age. It can be classified in two ways, either, according to its temporal progression, or according to its cause.

Transplantation at a Glance, First Edition. Menna Clatworthy, Christopher Watson, Michael Allison and John Dark.

Classification by temporal progression

The rapid onset of renal failure over a period of days or weeks is termed 'acute renal failure' or 'acute kidney injury' (AKI), whereas a decline in GFR occurring over months to years is termed 'chronic renal failure' or 'chronic kidney disease' (CKD).

Classification of renal failure by cause

The cause of renal failure can be classified using the terms:
- pre-renal
- renal
- post-renal.

These indicate the anatomical site at which the aetiological factor is acting. For example, systemic hypotension due to blood loss will compromise the renal blood flow and is a 'pre-renal' cause of renal failure. In contrast, inflammatory disease of the glomerulus (glomerulonephritis, GN) is a 'renal' cause of renal failure. Enlargement of the prostate causing obstruction to the outflow of urine is a 'post-renal' cause of renal failure.

Acute kidney injury

The most common cause of AKI is pre-renal failure, which if left untreated will progress to acute tubular necrosis (ATN). ATN occurs if there is persistent hypotension/hypovolaemia and/or exposure to nephrotoxins or sepsis. It is the cause of 60–80% of cases of AKI. ATN is quite common because the renal tubular blood supply is relatively precarious, so that any drop in blood pressure (secondary to hypovolaemia or reduced peripheral vascular resistance as seen in sepsis) can lead to tubular ischaemia. This is a direct result of the anatomical arrangement of the blood supply, which comes to the tubules only after it has passed through the glomerular capillary bed. Thus, there is always relative hypoxia in the renal medulla compared with the cortex. When the mean arterial pressure falls, there will be a reduced blood flow into the glomerulus via the afferent arteriole and a consequent fall in GFR. This prompts an increase in vasoconstriction in the efferent glomerular arteriole in an attempt to maintain GFR, which will further compromise the blood supply to the medulla, leading to increased hypoxia and tubular ischaemia. Tubular cells are also very metabolically active, with a number of energy-requiring electrolyte pumps. All of these factors contribute to susceptibility to ATN.

Histologically, ATN is manifest as ragged, dying tubular cells, which lose their nuclei and begin to slough off into the tubular lumen. Patients with pre-renal failure should be given fluid to restore intravascular volume and nephrotoxins (non-steroidal anti-inflammatory drugs [NSAIDs], gentamicin or ACEi) should be removed. ATN usually recovers spontaneously, although the patient may temporarily require renal replacement therapy (RRT). Some patients sustain irreversible tubular atrophy and a degree of chronic kidney damage.

Other causes of AKI include GNs (5–10%), obstruction (5–10%), and acute tubulointerstitial nephritis (TIN) (<5%).

GNs are named according to the appearance of the renal biopsy. For example, in minimal change GN there is no abnormality in the biopsy when viewed with a light microscope; in membranous GN there is thickening of the glomerular basement membrane. IgA nephropathy is characterised by the deposition of IgA in the mesangium, etc. Some primary and secondary GNs commonly present with an acute decline in renal function, while others commonly result in CKD (see below). GNs presenting as AKI include:
- Primary – pauci-immune crescentic GN, anti-glomerular basement membrane disease (Goodpasture's disease).
- Secondary – lupus nephritis, antineutrophil cytoplasmic antibody (ANCA)-associated vasculitis.

Patients with acute GN may require RRT as well as treatment for the underlying disease (e.g. immunosuppression +/– plasma exchange). The success of these treatments is variable; some patients partially regain renal function while others become permanently dialysis-dependent.

Acute TIN often occurs as the result of an 'allergic reaction' to medications, both prescription drugs such as proton pump inhibitors or antibiotics, and herbal remedies. Renal biopsy demonstrates an intense lymphocytic infiltrate in the interstitium, including numerous eosinophils. Management involves removal of the likely causative agent and the administration of oral corticosteroids to reduce renal inflammation. This usually results in the resolution of acute inflammation, but some patients are left with irreversible interstitial fibrosis and tubular atrophy, which may contribute to the subsequent development of CKD.

CKD

CKD can be completely asymptomatic until its very terminal stages. Eventually anaemia (manifest as tiredness or even congestive cardiac failure), uraemia (resulting in nausea, reduced appetite and confusion), phosphate build-up (leading to itchiness) and/or severe hypertension (causing headache or blurred vision) may prompt the patient to seek medical attention, where a routine blood test reveals high urea and creatinine due to a reduced GFR.

In contrast to AKI, where pre-renal and post-renal causes predominate, the causes of CKD tend to be renal in origin. These include:
- diabetes mellitus with associated diabetic nephropathy
- hypertensive nephropathy
- obstructive uropathy (often secondary to prostatic hypertrophy)
- chronic primary GN, e.g. IgA nephropathy or focal segmental glomerulosclerosis (FSGS)
- chronic secondary GN, e.g. lupus nephritis
- adult polycystic kidney disease (APKD)
- chronic pyelonephritis
- renovascular disease.

CKD is classified into different stages according to the patient's GFR and the presence of urine dipstick abnormalities. These have allowed the development of management guidelines for patients with stable CKD, and facilitate the provision of consistent care.

Diseases that recur in the transplant

A number of causes of renal failure may reoccur in the allograft. These include:
- structural problems – bladder outflow obstruction
- renal calculi
- urinary tract infections with associated chronic pyelonephritis
- primary GNs – IgA, FSGS, mesangiocapillary glomerulonephritis (MCGN)
- secondary GNs – ANCA-associated vasculitis, lupus nephritis, diabetic nephropathy.

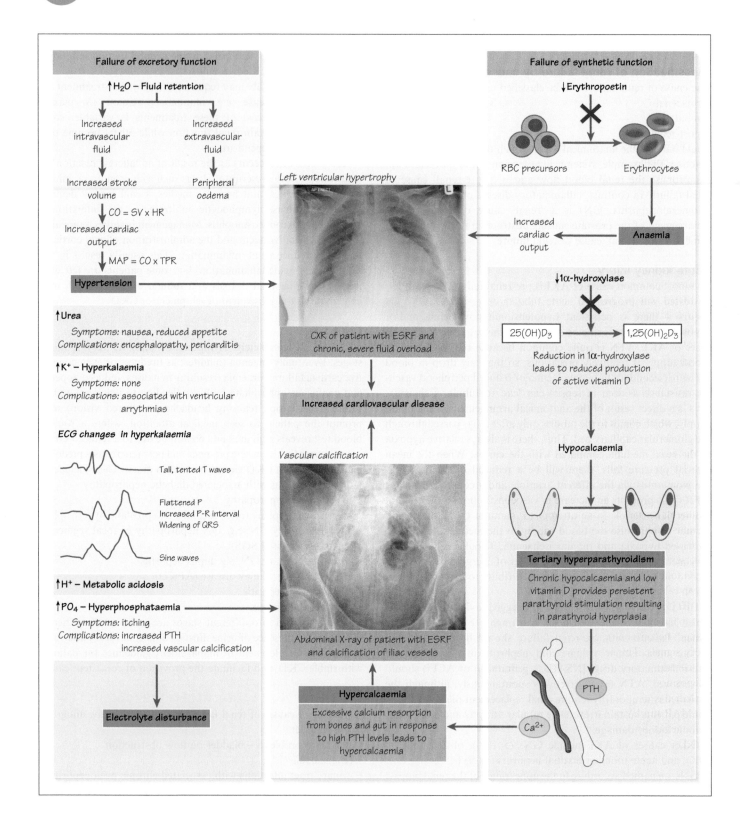

Failure of excretory function

↑H₂O – Fluid retention

Increased intravascular fluid → Increased stroke volume → ↓CO = SV × HR → Increased cardiac output → ↓MAP = CO × TPR → **Hypertension**

Increased extravascular fluid → Peripheral oedema

↑Urea
Symptoms: nausea, reduced appetite
Complications: encephalopathy, pericarditis

↑K⁺ – Hyperkalaemia
Symptoms: none
Complications: associated with ventricular arrythmias

ECG changes in hyperkalaemia
— Tall, tented T waves
— Flattened P
Increased P-R interval
Widening of QRS
— Sine waves

↑H⁺ – Metabolic acidosis

↑PO₄ – Hyperphosphataemia
Symptoms: itching
Complications: increased PTH
increased vascular calcification

Electrolyte disturbance

Left ventricular hypertrophy

CXR of patient with ESRF and chronic, severe fluid overload

Increased cardiovascular disease

Vascular calcification

Abdominal X-ray of patient with ESRF and calcification of iliac vessels

Hypercalcaemia
Excessive calcium resorption from bones and gut in response to high PTH levels leads to hypercalcaemia

Failure of synthetic function

↓Erythropoetin

RBC precursors ✗→ Erythrocytes

Increased cardiac output ← **Anaemia**

↓1α-hydroxylase

25(OH)D₃ ✗→ 1,25(OH)₂D₃

Reduction in 1α-hydroxylase leads to reduced production of active vitamin D

Hypocalcaemia

Tertiary hyperparathyroidism
Chronic hypocalcaemia and low vitamin D provides persistent parathyroid stimulation resulting in parathyroid hyperplasia

PTH

Ca²⁺

Transplantation at a Glance, First Edition. Menna Clatworthy, Christopher Watson, Michael Allison and John Dark.

Normally functioning kidneys accomplish a number of important tasks.

1 Control of water balance.

2 Control of electrolyte balance.

3 Control of blood pressure (through both control of water and electrolyte balance and production of renin).

4 Control of acid-base balance.

5 Excretion of water-soluble waste.

6 The production of active vitamin D (though the action of 1α hydroxylase) and hence control of calcium-phosphate metabolism.

7 The production of erythropoietin (EPO), and hence control of haemoglobin concentration.

In patients with ESRF, one or more of the above functions cannot be performed, resulting in a number of complications.

Failure of renal excretory functions

Control of water balance

As tubular function declines, the kidney retains fluid, resulting in an expansion in intravascular volume and an increase in venous return. Since mean arterial pressure (MAP) is dependent on cardiac output (CO) and total peripheral resistance (TPR), and CO is affected by stroke volume and hence venous return, the principal effect of fluid retention is hypertension. Patients with CKD and even those on dialysis are often chronically volume overloaded. The resulting hypertension places strain on the left ventricle, leading to left ventricular hypertrophy (LVH) and eventually LV dilatation.

Control of electrolyte balance

Patients fail to excrete potassium appropriately, leading to hyperkalaemia, which can result in life-threatening cardiac arrhythmias. Sodium retention contributes to fluid overload and hypertension.

Accumulation of phosphate leads to the release of two hormones that would normally increase phosphate excretion by the kidneys: parathyroid hormone (PTH, released by the parathyroid glands) and fibroblast growth factor 23 (FGF23, released by bone cells). Unfortunately, FGF23 inhibits 1α-hydroxylase activity, worsening vitamin D deficiency (see below). Low vitamin D levels lead to a further increase in PTH, because parathyroid cells sense both calcium and vitamin D. The end result is a spiralling increase in PTH, releasing calcium from bone and increasing phosphate, establishing a vicious cycle. If left untreated, the parathyroid glands become enlarged and stop responding to the normal inhibitory signals. This leads to hypercalcaemia and is termed tertiary hyperparathyroidism. Chronic hypercalcaemia results in calcium deposition in soft tissues and arteries. Arteries can become heavily calcified and stiff, leading to decreased compliance and an increase in MAP and LVH. Calcium deposition is enhanced by hyperphosphataemia and the metabolic acidosis that often accompanies CKD.

Control of acid-base balance

The kidneys normally excrete the daily acid load generated by amino acid metabolism. As renal function declines, patients develop a progressive metabolic acidosis. Chronic acidosis can promote renal bone disease (see below) and leads to muscle wasting and malnutrition.

Excretion of soluble waste products

The kidneys are responsible for excreting most soluble waste products, including urea. In CKD, urea levels rise, resulting in a loss of appetite and nausea. At higher levels, uraemia may be associated with pericarditis and encephalopathy.

Failure of renal synthetic functions

Activity of 1-α hydroxylase

Native vitamin D (cholecalciferol) is hydroxylated first by the liver to 25-hydroxy vitamin D, and then by the kidneys to the active hormone 1, 25 dihydroxyvitamin D3 (calcitriol). Low circulating calcitriol levels are characteristic of patients with kidney failure, due to loss of the activating enzyme 1-α hydroxylase. Calcitriol is central to calcium homeostasis: its deficiency in CKD leads to a reduction in intestinal calcium absorption, hypocalcaemia and impaired mineralisation of bone, manifesting as 'renal rickets' in children and osteomalacia in adults. Bone disease in CKD may also be due to high turnover due to high PTH, or low turnover due to over-suppressed PTH.

Erythropoietin production

EPO is produced by peritubular cells and acts on erythroid precursors within the bone marrow, stimulating proliferation and maturation. When the GFR falls to <50 ml/min, a reduction in EPO production may be observed, resulting in anaemia. Anaemia in CKD patients is exacerbated by impaired intestinal absorption of iron and reduced iron intake (due to nausea secondary to uraemia). Anaemia can lead to an increase in cardiac output and may exacerbate LV dysfunction. Prior to the introduction of recombinant EPO, anaemia was a major cause of morbidity and mortality in patients with ESRF due to associated cardiovascular complications.

Morbidity and mortality of patients with CKD/ESRF

Patients with ESRF have a significantly increased mortality compared with the general population. This is mainly due to an increase in atherosclerosis and vascular calcification, which result in accelerated coronary artery disease, peripheral vascular disease and cerebrovascular accidents. These complications may significantly impact their fitness for transplantation.

Patients reaching ESRF are also susceptible to additional complications related to the provision of renal replacement therapy (RRT), as detailed in Chapter 23.

23 Dialysis and its complications

Types of dialysis

Haemodialysis
• 3–4 hrs, 3 x /week
• Most patients travel to dialysis unit
• Requires vascular access:

(a) Tunnelled central line   (b) Arteriovenous fistula

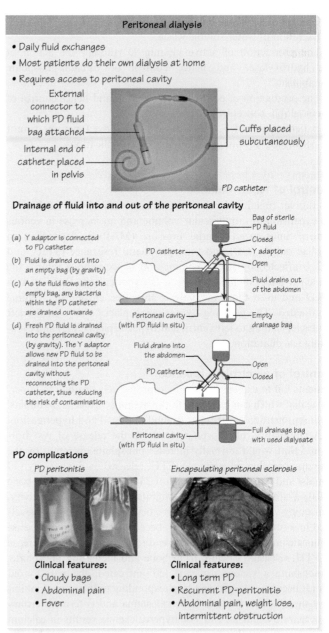

Principles of dialysis

From patient → To patient

Solute   Blood flow

High blood solute concentration   Low blood solute concentration

Semi-permeable dialysis membrane

Net direction of solute and water movement

Direction of dialysate flow (converse direction to blood flow to optimise maintenance of solute gradient)

HD complications

- Line-associated complications:
  – Infection (tunnel/endocarditis)
  – Central vein thrombosis
  – Central vein stenosis
- AVF-associated complications:
  – Steal
  – Thrombosis
- General HD complications:
  – Increased cardiovascular disease

Peritoneal dialysis
• Daily fluid exchanges
• Most patients do their own dialysis at home
• Requires access to peritoneal cavity

External connector to which PD fluid bag attached

Internal end of catheter placed in pelvis

Cuffs placed subcutaneously

PD catheter

Drainage of fluid into and out of the peritoneal cavity

(a) Y adaptor is connected to PD catheter

(b) Fluid is drained out into an empty bag (by gravity)

(c) As the fluid flows into the empty bag, any bacteria within the PD catheter are drained outwards

(d) Fresh PD fluid is drained into the peritoneal cavity (by gravity). The Y adaptor allows new PD fluid to be drained into the peritoneal cavity without reconnecting the PD catheter, thus reducing the risk of contamination

Bag of sterile PD fluid
Closed
Y adaptor
Open
PD catheter
Fluid drains out of the abdomen
Peritoneal cavity (with PD fluid in situ)
Empty drainage bag

Fluid drains into the abdomen
PD catheter
Open
Closed
Peritoneal cavity (with PD fluid in situ)
Full drainage bag with used dialysate

PD complications

PD peritonitis   Encapsulating peritoneal sclerosis

Clinical features:
- Cloudy bags
- Abdominal pain
- Fever

Clinical features:
- Long term PD
- Recurrent PD-peritonitis
- Abdominal pain, weight loss, intermittent obstruction

Limitations of dialysis

(a) Lifestyle and survival limitations on dialysis

Fluid – 3 cups/day (750 ml)

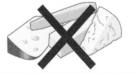 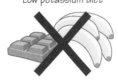

Low phosphate diet   Low potassium diet

(b) Survival on dialysis based on renal registry data (1997–2005)

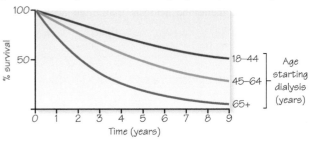

% survival vs Time (years)

18–44
45–64
65+

Age starting dialysis (years)

Transplantation at a Glance, First Edition. Menna Clatworthy, Christopher Watson, Michael Allison and John Dark.

Once a patient's glomerular filtration rate (GFR) falls below 15 ml/min/1.73m^2 they require renal replacement therapy (RRT), either haemodialysis (HD), peritoneal dialysis (PD) or transplantation. Both haemo- and peritoneal dialysis are associated with specific complications, in addition to the general complications associated with ESRF.

Haemodialysis complications

Complications related to vascular access

Vascular access is required to administer HD. For acute HD, this may be achieved using a temporary central dialysis catheter (which can be used for a week or so). Temporary catheters are often placed in the femoral vein, although this may compromise the vessel for future use during transplantation.

In the medium term, vascular access can be provided via a tunnelled central catheter, which can last for a number of months. The main complication of tunnelled lines is infection, including:
- exit site infections
- tunnel infections
- infective endocarditis.

These are commonly caused by skin-colonising staphylococci. The presence of active infection precludes the patient from transplantation, as the addition of immunosuppression may be life threatening.

Other line-related complications include the following.
- Line insertion-related – pneumothorax and/or vascular injury.
- Thrombosis – a large thrombus can sometimes form on the tip of the catheter, which can become infected. These often form in the right atrium, and their removal may require open cardiac surgery.
- Central vein stenosis – particularly with subclavian vein catheters and catheters that remain in situ for prolonged periods (months or even years).

For patients on HD, the vascular access of choice is an arteriovenous fistula (AVF). These are formed by joining the radial or brachial artery with the cephalic vein and they provide vascular access without the presence of indwelling catheter (therefore lowering the risk of infection). Ideally, the cephalic and brachial veins of either arm should not be used for cannulation or venepuncture in patients approaching ESRF in anticipation of their later use for AVF formation.

Occlusion/thrombosis of an AVF can occur if the patient becomes hypotensive on dialysis, if they are hypercoagulable or have a stenosis of the draining vein; thrombosis is also common following transplantation, either due to peri-operative hypotension or the removal of the uraemic inhibitory effect on platelet aggregation. The AV fistula itself may become aneurysmal or steal blood from the circulation, rendering the distal limb ischaemic.

Other complications

To achieve adequate RRT, most patients will need to undergo haemodialysis for 3–4 hours, three times a week. This involves a journey to the local dialysis centre, which may be some distance from the patient's home. If they are reliant on 'hospital transport', the whole process can take the best part of a day, making it difficult for the patient to maintain full-time employment.

Fluid balance can be a particular problem in anuric patients on dialysis, many of whom struggle to restrict their fluid intake to the necessary 500–750 ml/24 hours. Such patients often need to have 2–3 litres removed during their dialysis session, which can result in peri-dialysis hypotension and leave them feeling totally exhausted.

In summary, haemodialysis can replace some of the functions of the kidney, but carries specific morbidities and imposes significant restrictions on a patient's quality of life.

Peritoneal dialysis complications

PD involves the placement of a catheter into the peritoneal cavity. This is tunnelled underneath the skin to limit the translocation of infectious organisms from the surface into the peritoneum. The catheter is used to instil 1–2 litres of dialysate into the abdominal cavity via one of two methods.

1 *Manual method: continuous ambulatory peritoneal dialysis (CAPD).* The patient manually connects a bag of PD fluid to the dialysis catheter via a transfer set and instils fluid into the peritoneal cavity using gravity. The fluid is then drained out (again using gravity) after a dwell period of several hours. This procedure is repeated three or four times a day.

2 *Automated method: automated peritoneal dialysis (APD).* This refers to all forms of PD employing a mechanical device to assist in the delivery and drainage of the dialysate, usually overnight. The main advantage of APD is that it allows freedom from all procedures during the day.

The PD fluid needs to be similar in composition to interstitial fluid, and hypertonic to plasma in order to achieve fluid removal. Glucose is used as an osmotic agent and solutions of differing strengths are used, depending on how much ultrafiltration (fluid removal) is required.

The main complication of PD is the development of infection, ('PD peritonitis'). Patients usually present with abdominal pain and the drainage of cloudy PD fluid from the abdomen. Gram-positive organisms cause up to 75% of all episodes of peritonitis, mainly *Staphylococcus epidermidis* or, more seriously, *S. aureus.* The latter can be associated with a more severe illness, which may be life threatening. Treatment is with intraperitoneal and systemic antibiotics; catheter removal may be required. Patients with active PD peritonitis should be temporarily suspended from the transplant waiting list until resolution of infection.

Encapsulating peritoneal sclerosis (EPS) is a well-recognised, although uncommon, complication of long-term PD, occurring in 1–5% of patients. Macroscopic changes in the peritoneum can be seen after relatively short periods of PD, particularly 'tanning' of the peritoneum. Patients who remain on PD for a number of years can develop more extensive peritoneal thickening, with superimposed fibrous tissue encasing the bowel. Clinical features include vomiting and distension (secondary to bowel obstruction), blood-stained effluent and ultrafiltration failure. Radiological features include peritoneal thickening and calcification, with the development of the so-called 'abdominal cocoon'. Risk factors include multiple episodes of peritonitis and long duration of dialysis. The main treatment is to avoid EPS by stopping PD when dialysis adequacy declines, or when evidence of peritoneal sclerosis is noted on CT. EPS, if present, should be treated before listing for transplantation; malnourishment due to EPS is a contraindication to transplantation. EPS can present post-transplantation.

Mortality on dialysis

The complications of ESRF, together with those associated with dialysis, have a significant impact on patient survival. On average, a 50-year-old commencing haemodialysis has a 50% 5-year survival. This can be significantly improved by transplantation.

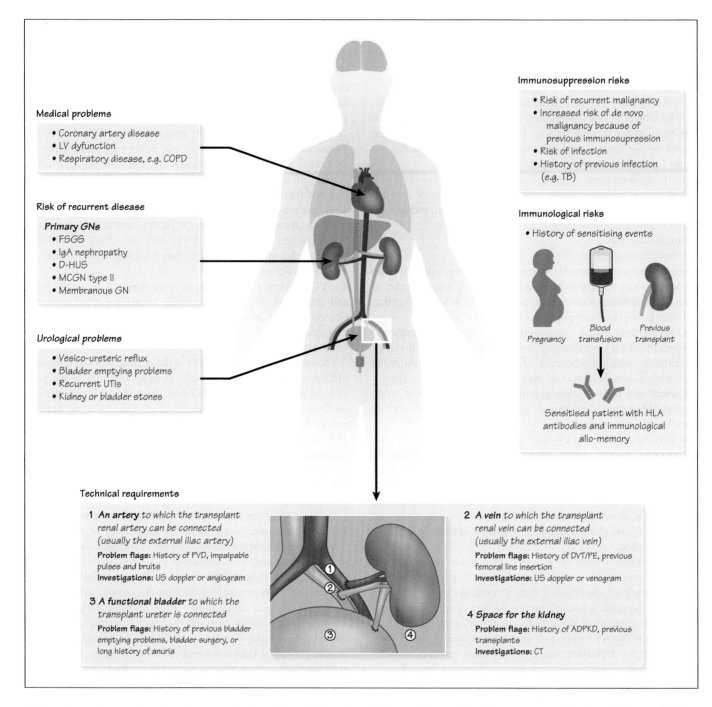

Medical problems

- Coronary artery disease
- LV dyfunction
- Respiratory disease, e.g. COPD

Risk of recurrent disease

Primary GNs
- FSGS
- IgA nephropathy
- D-HUS
- MCGN type II
- Membranous GN

Urological problems

- Vesico-ureteric reflux
- Bladder emptying problems
- Recurrent UTIs
- Kidney or bladder stones

Immunosuppression risks

- Risk of recurrent malignancy
- Increased risk of de novo malignancy because of previous immunosupression
- Risk of infection
- History of previous infection (e.g. TB)

Immunological risks

- History of sensitising events

Pregnancy / Blood transfusion / Previous transplant

Sensitised patient with HLA antibodies and immunological allo-memory

Technical requirements

1 An artery to which the transplant renal artery can be connected (usually the external iliac artery)
Problem flags: History of PVD, impalpable pulses and bruits
Investigations: US doppler or angiogram

3 A functional bladder to which the transplant ureter is connected
Problem flags: History of previous bladder emptying problems, bladder surgery, or long history of anuria

2 A vein to which the transplant renal vein can be connected (usually the external iliac vein)
Problem flags: History of DVT/PE, previous femoral line insertion
Investigations: US doppler or venogram

4 Space for the kidney
Problem flags: History of ADPKD, previous transplants
Investigations: CT

Although renal transplantation improves both quality of life and survival, it involves a significant investment of health resources and the use of an organ with a limited supply. It is therefore of utmost importance that the potential transplant recipient is carefully assessed, both to avoid unnecessary exposure to the risks of a general anaesthetic and to ensure appropriate use of a precious resource. To this end, every potential transplant recipient is assessed by taking a careful history, performing a thorough examination and undertaking a number of investigations.

The transplant work-up must answer five questions.

1 Does the patient have any medical problems which put them at risk of operative morbidity/mortality?
Patients with CKD are at increased risk of coronary, cerebral and peripheral vascular disease, and should be assessed for a past or current history of cardiac problems (e.g. angina, myocardial infarction, rheumatic fever), strokes or peripheral vascular disease (claudication/amputation). Risk factors assessed include family history, smoking history and a history of diabetes mellitus or hypercholesterolaemia. Smoking is also associated with the development of chronic obstructive pulmonary disease (COPD). A

Transplantation at a Glance, First Edition. Menna Clatworthy, Christopher Watson, Michael Allison and John Dark.

good screening question to assess general cardiorespiratory fitness is to ask how far the patient can walk; a good test is to make them walk.

Dialysis patients are frequently oligo-anuric and often struggle to restrict their fluid intake. This leads to chronic volume overload and hypertension, resulting in left ventricular hypertrophy (LVH) or dysfunction. Patient who require 3–4 litres of fluid to be removed at each dialysis session frequently develop such cardiac problems.

CKD is also associated with tertiary hyperparathyroidism and hypercalcaemia, which increases the risk of vascular and valvular calcification, particularly the aortic valve.

Examination should pay particular attention to cardiovascular signs: pulse rhythm and volume, signs of volume overload (elevated jugular venous pressure [JVP], peripheral and pulmonary oedema), signs of LVH (hyperdynamic apex beat) or LV dilatation (displaced apex beat) and signs of valvular heart disease (particularly the ejection systolic murmur of calcific aortic stenosis). The chest should be assessed for signs of COPD (hyperinflation, reduced expansion, wheeze) or for pleural effusions which may occur in patients on peritoneal dialysis.

Cardiorespiratory investigations include an electrocardiogram (ECG), a chest radiograph, a cardiac stress test (an exercise tolerance test or an isotope perfusion study) and an echocardiogram (to assess LV function). If these are abnormal, then the patient may need further cardiological assessment, including coronary angiography.

2 Does the patient have any conditions that make them technically difficult to transplant?

There are four basic technical requirements for implantation of a kidney.

• *An artery* (usually the external iliac artery), to which the transplant renal artery will be anastomosed. Severe vascular disease can make the arterial anastomosis difficult, therefore all of the patient's lower limb pulses should be carefully assessed during examination, including auscultation of the femoral arteries and aortic bifurcation for bruits, as a surrogate for iliac artery disease. Duplex imaging is indicated if any abnormality is detected or suspected.

• *A vein* (usually the external iliac vein), to which the transplant renal vein will be anastomosed. A history of venous thromboembolic disease, particularly clots in the lower limb veins, should be sought; a transplant should not be placed above a limb where a thrombosis has occurred previously. Patients on chronic haemodialysis may have had numerous lines inserted into their femoral veins, which can lead to stenosis and thrombosis. Look for collaterals, cutaneous signs of venous hypertension and oedema, which may be associated with venous compromise. Duplex imaging or percutaneous venography may be required.

• *A bladder*, to which the transplant ureter will be anastomosed. A history of urological problems, including congenital bladder malformations or reflux, is of relevance. If these issues are not resolved prior to transplantation, then they may recur and damage the transplanted kidney. Patients who have had ESRF for a number of years often have negligible urine output and a small, shrunken bladder, which is difficult to find intra-operatively and will only hold small volumes of urine post transplant. Some patients need a neobladder fashioned from a segment of their ileum (a urostomy).

• *Space for the kidney*. Some patients with polycystic kidney disease have grossly enlarged native kidneys that extend into the lower abdomen and may require removal prior to transplantation. In addition, patients with an elevated body mass index (BMI) may be technically difficult to transplant, due to lack of space for the graft and reduced ease of access to the vessels. Therefore, most centres will not list patients for transplantation unless the BMI is $<35\,kg/m^2$.

3 Is the patient at increased risk of the immunological complications of transplantation?

The immune system remains a significant barrier to transplantation in patients with pre-formed antibodies to non-self human leucocyte antigens (HLA). This usually occurs as a result of a sensitising event, for example blood transfusion, pregnancy (particularly by multiple partners), or previous renal transplants or other allografts (e.g. skin grafts). The frequency of such events should be ascertained.

4 Is the patient at increased risk of immunosuppression-associated complications?

Patients with ESRF secondary to a primary or secondary glomerulonephritis (e.g. IgA, vasculitis or lupus) have frequently been treated with immunosuppressants. This includes the use of toxic agents, such as cyclophosphamide, or biological agents, including alemtuzumab or rituximab. Heavy immunosuppression should be avoided in such patients post-transplant, particularly the use of lymphocyte-depleting agents such as anti-thymocyte globulin (ATG), which may place them at high risk of infectious complications.

Immunosuppression also increases the risk of developing a *de novo* cancer (particularly oncovirus-associated malignancies), and enhances the progression of existing cancers. Thus, most centres would agree that patients with a history of malignancy must be cancer-free for at least 5 years prior to transplantation.

5 Is the patient at risk of recurrent disease in their transplant?

Some pathologies that cause CKD can recur in the transplant and reduce its long-term function and survival. A number of glomerulonephritides can affect the graft (e.g. IgA nephropathy and focal segmental glomerulosclerosis [FSGS]). In the case of FSGS, the patient may develop recurrent disease immediately post transplant (usually evidenced by heavy proteinuria). This is sometimes amenable to treatment with plasma exchange, therefore it is important to recognise this risk and carefully monitor the patient post transplant. If a patient has developed rapidly progressive, recurrent disease in a transplant kidney, then this is a relative contraindication to re-transplantation.

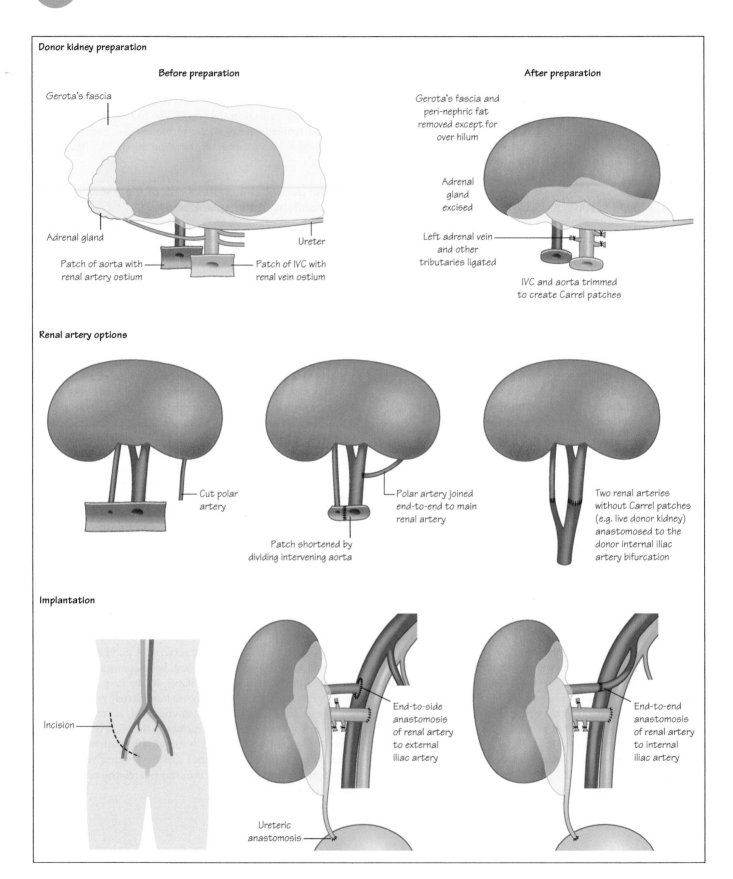

Donor kidney preparation

Before preparation

Gerota's fascia

Adrenal gland

Patch of aorta with
renal artery ostium

Ureter

Patch of IVC with
renal vein ostium

After preparation

Gerota's fascia and
peri-nephric fat
removed except for
over hilum

Adrenal
gland
excised

Left adrenal vein
and other
tributaries ligated

IVC and aorta trimmed
to create Carrel patches

Renal artery options

Cut polar
artery

Polar artery joined
end-to-end to main
renal artery

Patch shortened by
dividing intervening aorta

Two renal arteries
without Carrel patches
(e.g. live donor kidney)
anastomosed to the
donor internal iliac
artery bifurcation

Implantation

Incision

End-to-side
anastomosis
of renal artery
to external
iliac artery

Ureteric
anastomosis

End-to-end
anastomosis
of renal artery
to internal
iliac artery

Transplantation at a Glance, First Edition. Menna Clatworthy, Christopher Watson, Michael Allison and John Dark.

The donor kidney
Renal anatomy and anomalies
Most kidneys have a single artery and vein, although the incidence of multiple vessels is significant (10–20%). Multiple arteries usually arise close to each other, although a lower pole artery sometimes arises from the iliac artery instead of the aorta; others may take origin anywhere along the abdominal aorta, although most arise at or just below the origin of the superior mesenteric artery. Multiple veins may also occur, more commonly on the right than the left; when they do occur on the left the caudal vein sometimes passes behind the aorta; the left renal vein invariably passes in front.

Double ureters may also occur, although in the vast majority of cases only a single ureter is present.

Preparation of the donor kidney
When a deceased donor kidney is removed it is generally removed with a wide margin of surrounding tissue, including peri-renal fat and fascia, to preserve any possible anomalous vessels. This is not the case with live donor kidneys, where the vascular anatomy is usually known before nephrectomy and it is undesirable to remove too much extra tissue. Before implantation the deceased donor kidney is inspected for damage, either caused during retrieval or as a consequence of the catecholamine storm in the donor. Typical injuries are tears in the intima (the lining) of the artery, a consequence of either traction on the artery or donor hypertension when coning occurs.

Finally, the inferior vena cava (IVC) and aorta around the origins of both renal vein and artery are trimmed to produce Carrel patches to facilitate implantation.

Implantation
Patient preparation
In order to monitor fluid status post operatively a central venous catheter is usually placed at the time of transplantation, in addition to the other peri-operative monitoring.

A urinary catheter is also placed, and connected to a bag of normal saline containing a blue dye (e.g. methylene blue) or antibiotic or both. This allows the bladder to be inflated so it can be easily located during surgery, and the blue dye permits confirmation by the surgeon that it is the bladder that he/she has opened and not the peritoneum or a loop of bowel.

Surgical procedure
The donor kidney is implanted in one or other iliac fossa, with the right side being generally preferred to the left since the iliac vessels are nearer to the surface. Dissection extends through the muscles but remains outside the peritoneal cavity. By keeping extraperitoneal and away from the intestine, the patient can resume eating and drinking soon after surgery. Extraperitoneal placement also has advantages later when it comes to taking a biopsy of the kidney, since any bleeding that may follow is relatively contained, rather than filling the entire peritoneal cavity.

The peritoneum is displaced medially to expose the external iliac artery and vein, the blood vessels that take blood to and from the leg. They are surrounded by lymphatic tissue and this is dissected free; it is this process that may predispose to lymphocoele formation post-operatively.

Most deceased donor kidneys are implanted with the renal artery anastomosed to the recipient's external iliac artery, and renal vein to the external iliac vein. This technique was first developed in Paris in the early 1950s, and was the placement copied by Murray when he performed his first transplant in 1954. The lower pole of the kidney now lies in proximity to the bladder, facilitating the ureteric anastomosis. The ureter is anastomosed to the dome of the bladder and, in most transplant units, a double J stent, a small plastic tube, is inserted to splint the anastomosis; this is removed cystoscopically 6 weeks later.

Where there is no Carrel patch on the artery, such as with kidneys from live donors, the renal artery may be joined end-to-end to the internal iliac artery. Multiple renal arteries may be joined to the divisions of the recipient's own internal iliac artery on the back table before implantation.

Special considerations
Multiple arteries and veins

There is a network of veins within the kidney, so in general the smaller of two veins can be tied off. This is not the case for the arterial supply, which is end-artery and needs to be preserved. Where possible the multiple arteries are brought close together onto a single patch to make implantation easier; cut polar vessels are implanted into the side of the main artery or, if large, implanted separately.

Children
Transplanting kidneys into small children is done at a few specialist centres. Generally live donor or young adult deceased donor kidneys are used. For small children, implantation is on to the aorta and IVC, usually intra-peritoneal, rather than to the external iliac vessels, which would be too small.

Paediatric kidney transplantation has implications regarding fluid balance – the blood volume of an adult kidney may be half the circulating volume of a small child, so careful and experienced anaesthetic support is essential.

Ileal conduits

Some patients have a non-functioning bladder or have previously undergone a cystectomy. In order to provide a urinary reservoir a short segment of ileum is isolated and one end brought to the surface as a stoma. This urostomy (or ileal conduit) acts as a bladder; the transplant ureter is implanted at its base. A stoma appliance is placed over the urostomy to collect the urine.

Transplant outcomes
Renal transplantation significantly improves patient survival compared with dialysis. Current UK 1-year, 5-year and 10-year patient and graft survival following a first kidney transplant are summarised below.

Donor type	Survival	1 year	5 year	10 year
Live donor kidney	Graft	96%	90%	78%
	Patient	99%	96%	89%
Deceased DBD donor kidney	Graft	93%	83%	67%
	Patient	97%	88%	71%

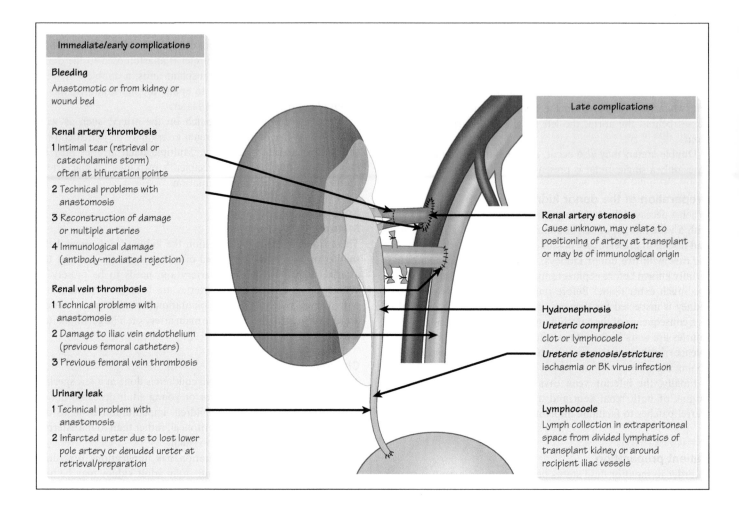

Immediate/early complications

Bleeding
Anastomotic or from kidney or wound bed

Renal artery thrombosis
1 Intimal tear (retrieval or catecholamine storm) often at bifurcation points
2 Technical problems with anastomosis
3 Reconstruction of damage or multiple arteries
4 Immunological damage (antibody-mediated rejection)

Renal vein thrombosis
1 Technical problems with anastomosis
2 Damage to iliac vein endothelium (previous femoral catheters)
3 Previous femoral vein thrombosis

Urinary leak
1 Technical problem with anastomosis
2 Infarcted ureter due to lost lower pole artery or denuded ureter at retrieval/preparation

Late complications

Renal artery stenosis
Cause unknown, may relate to positioning of artery at transplant or may be of immunological origin

Hydronephrosis
Ureteric compression:
clot or lymphocoele
Ureteric stenosis/stricture:
ischaemia or BK virus infection

Lymphocoele
Lymph collection in extraperitoneal space from divided lymphatics of transplant kidney or around recipient iliac vessels

Post-transplant surgical complications usually present in the first days to weeks following transplantation. They can be divided into three broad categories:
• vascular complications
• ureteric complications
• wound complications.

Vascular complications
Renal artery thrombosis
This is a rare (<1% of transplants) and usually catastrophic complication. Endothelial damage during brain death and retrieval surgery may predispose to thrombosis, but most are due to technical complications with the anastomosis. Patients usually present in the first week post-transplant with a rapid decline in graft function and anuria. Diagnosis may be delayed in patients with post-transplant acute tubular necrosis (ATN), where these features are not discriminatory, or who have a good urine output from their own kidneys. Doppler ultrasound demonstrates a lack of renal perfusion. The patient should be taken back to theatre immediately in an attempt to remove the clot and restore perfusion to the graft. This is rarely successful, and most commonly the graft has already infarcted necessitating transplant nephrectomy.

Renal vein thrombosis
Renal vein thrombosis is also uncommon, occurring in around 2–5% of transplants. As with arterial thrombosis, the patient presents with declining graft function and oligo-anuria in the early post-transplant period. Venous thrombosis may also cause graft swelling, pain, and macroscopic haematuria and rupture of the kidney. Treatment is by urgent thombectomy, but the prognosis is poor. A number of aetiological factors have been suggested, including damage to the vein during retrieval, poor anastomotic technique, post-operative hypotension and venous compression by haematoma or lymphocoele. Patients with a history of previous venous thromboembolism or a known thrombophilic tendency should be carefully monitored or prophylactically anticoagulated, as they are at increased risk of this complication.

Renal artery stenosis
Renal artery stenosis is far more common (~5%) than vascular thromboses and usually presents much later, at around 3 to 6 months post transplant. The stenosis usually occurs just beyond the arterial anastomosis. Clinical features include refractory hypertension, a gradual decline in renal function or a sharp decline following the introduction of ACE inhibitors. Examination may

Transplantation at a Glance, First Edition. Menna Clatworthy, Christopher Watson, Michael Allison and John Dark.

reveal a bruit over the graft, but this is relatively non-specific. The diagnosis is confirmed by angiography and treatment is percutaneous balloon angioplasty. Recurrence occurs in one-third of cases, requiring further angioplasty, stent insertion or even surgical intervention. Anastomotic renal artery stenosis occurs mainly in live donor transplants where no Carrel patch is present.

Ureteric complications

Urine leak

Urinary leaks usually present in the first days/weeks post transplant, often when the urinary catheter is removed. They mostly occur due to leakage at the site of anastomosis of donor ureter to bladder. It is either due to poor surgical technique or ureteric necrosis. The latter complication often results from over-enthusiastic stripping of the adventitial tissue from around the ureter during preparation for implantation. Patients present with discharge of fluid from the wound, which should be sent for biochemical analysis. Urine has a high creatinine and urea concentration (much higher than serum), whereas lymph has similar concentrations to serum. Anterograde pyelography/cystography allows identification of the leak.

Urine leaks are managed by decompressing the bladder by re-insertion of the urinary catheter. If a urinary stent is in situ, then catheterisation may be sufficient to limit the leak and allow healing to occur, although subsequent stricture formation is common. If there is no stent present, then percutaneous nephrostomy may be required as a prelude to surgical revision once the site of the leak is identified.

Ureteric obstruction

Ureteric obstruction may occur early post-transplant if a ureteric stent is not inserted. Causes include anastomotic strictures, luminal blood clot and extrinsic compression due to a lymphocoele. Obstruction presenting later (>3 months post transplant) is invariably due to a ureteric stricture, usually caused by ureteric ischaemia, possibly due to division of a small lower pole artery that supplied the ureter. Other causes of ureteric stenosis include infection (particularly BK virus infection) and rejection, particularly chronic rejection. Patients present with urinary leak (if obstruction occurs early) or a decline in renal function, and ultrasound demonstrates transplant hydronephrosis. Percutaneous nephrostomy

is required to decompress the kidney, and allows an anterograde nephrostogram to be performed, which will delineate the site and severity of the stricture. Short strictures (<2 cm) may be dilated and stented; more significant lesions require surgical intervention, with excision of the stricture and re-implantation of the ureter, or by anastomosis of the native ureter to the transplant ureter or collecting system.

Wound complications

Wound infection

Wound infections may be limited to the skin and subcutaneous tissue or may extend deeper into the fascia and muscle layers. More superficial infections present with erythema and swelling around the wound. Ultrasound may be useful in identifying deeper collections. Such patients may also have systemic symptoms such as fever. Treatment is with systemic antibiotics and surgical drainage of any collections.

Wound dehiscence

Superficial wound dehiscence may occur if there is infection or tension. Once infection is cleared, healing usually occurs spontaneously, and may be assisted by application of a vacuum dressing. Deeper dehiscence with disruption of the muscle layer is less common and requires surgical repair.

Lymphocoele

Lymphatics draining the transplant kidney, together with those surrounding the recipient's blood vessels, are divided as part of the transplant process. Lymph may leak from these and collect, forming a lymphocoele. Lymphocoeles are common, occurring in up to 20% of transplants but are mostly small (<3 cm) and asymptomatic. Larger collections may result in swelling or persistent discharge from the wound. Occasionally, collections may compress adjacent structures such as the ureter (resulting in hydronephrosis and transplant dysfunction) or the iliac vein (resulting in leg swelling or deep vein thrombosis). Small, asymptomatic lymphocoeles are left to resolve spontaneously. Larger collections require percutaneous drainage; if they recur (which is common), then surgical drainage is required, and involves making a window in the peritoneum to allow the lymphocoele to drain into the peritoneal cavity (a 'fenestration' procedure).

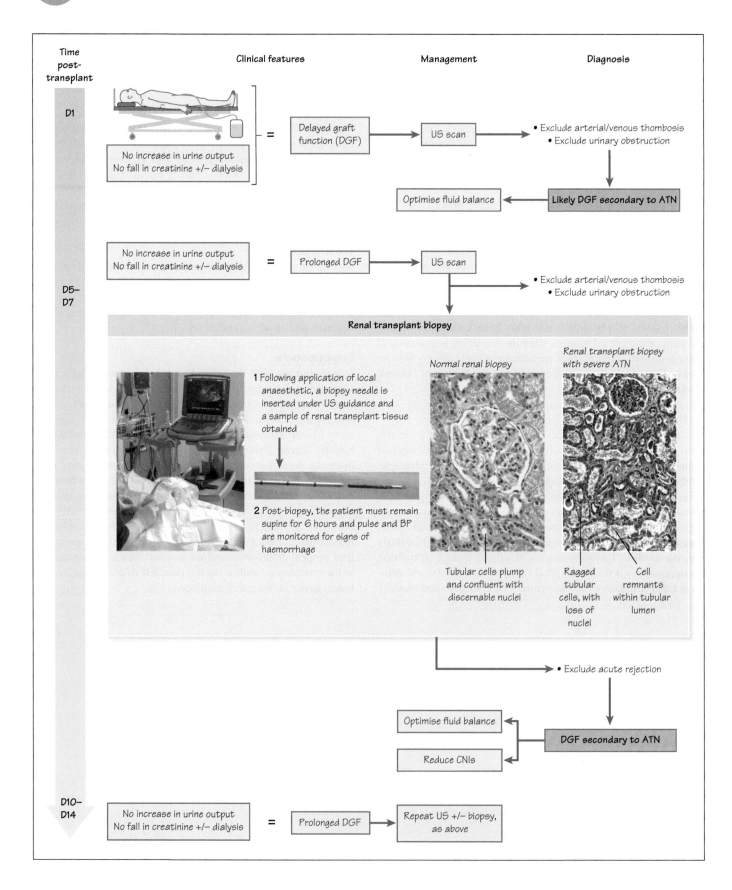

Time post-transplant

Clinical features

Management

Diagnosis

D1

No increase in urine output
No fall in creatinine +/− dialysis

= Delayed graft function (DGF) → US scan →
• Exclude arterial/venous thombosis
• Exclude urinary obstruction

Optimise fluid balance ← **Likely DGF secondary to ATN**

D5–D7

No increase in urine output
No fall in creatinine +/− dialysis

= Prolonged DGF → US scan
• Exclude arterial/venous thombosis
• Exclude urinary obstruction

Renal transplant biopsy

1 Following application of local anaesthetic, a biopsy needle is inserted under US guidance and a sample of renal transplant tissue obtained

2 Post-biopsy, the patient must remain supine for 6 hours and pulse and BP are monitored for signs of haemorrhage

Normal renal biopsy

Tubular cells plump and confluent with discernable nuclei

Renal transplant biopsy with severe ATN

Ragged tubular cells, with loss of nuclei

Cell remnants within tubular lumen

• Exclude acute rejection

Optimise fluid balance ←
Reduce CNIs ←
DGF secondary to ATN

D10–D14

No increase in urine output
No fall in creatinine +/− dialysis

= Prolonged DGF → Repeat US +/− biopsy, as above

Transplantation at a Glance, First Edition. Menna Clatworthy, Christopher Watson, Michael Allison and John Dark.

One of the most common complications occurring in the early post-transplant period is delayed graft function (DGF). Clinically, the patient is oliguric, fails to demonstrate an improvement in renal function, and will often require haemodialysis. It is important to note that allograft oliguria may not be obvious in renal transplant recipients who have significant residual native urine output. In such cases, the patient may return from theatre passing good volumes of urine (resulting from the intravenous fluids given intra-operatively), all of which originate from their own kidneys. It is therefore important to ascertain from the patient their usual urine output and interpret post-transplant urine output in light of this information.

Causes of DGF

The absence of graft function immediately post-transplant may be due to a number of causes:

1. Pre-renal causes:
   - arterial/venous thrombosis
   - systemic hypotension.
2. Renal causes:
   - acute tubular necrosis (ATN)
   - hyperacute rejection
   - aggressive recurrence of a primary GN.
3. Post-renal causes:
   - ureteric obstruction/leak
   - catheter blockage.

ATN is by far the most common cause of DGF, but this diagnosis should not be assumed, and other, more serious pathologies must be excluded.

Prevalence of DGF

DGF is relatively common, occurring in around 30% of kidneys donated after brainstem death (DBD), ≥50% of kidneys donated after circulatory death (DCD), but it is rare (<5%) in living donor kidneys.

Risk factors for post-transplant DGF

Donor factors

With the ever-increasing number of patients on the renal transplant waiting list, there has been an increasing use of less than ideal donor kidneys (that is, donors with increasing age or co-morbidities). This is inevitably associated with an increase in the rates of DGF. Donor risk factors for DGF include:

- higher donor age
- hypertension
- acute renal impairment
- treatment with nephrotoxins
- prolonged donor hypotension
- marked catecholamine storm during brainstem death.

Allograft factors

- Prolonged warm ischaemia.
- Prolonged cold ischaemia.
- Prolonged anastomosis time.

Recipient factors

- HLA-antibodies (sensitisation).
- Post-operative hypotension.

Diagnosis of post-transplant ATN

The diagnosis is usually one of exclusion. An ultrasound (US) scan allows the assessment of perfusion and venous drainage and whether there is dilatation of the pelvi-caliceal system (indicative of urinary obstruction). If these diagnoses are excluded, then a transplant biopsy should be performed in patients with persistent (>5 days) DGF to exclude rejection and to assess the severity of ATN and its recovery. As in native kidneys, transplant ATN is characterised by the presence of tatty-looking tubular cells, many of which lack nuclei and begin to slough off into the tubular lumen.

Performing a transplant renal biopsy

The main complication of renal transplant biopsy is haemorrhage. Therefore it is important to minimise the risk of this by ensuring the following.

1. The patient has normal clotting and platelets (>100 × 10^9/L). Most patients will be receiving low molecular weight heparin, but this should be omitted on the night before biopsy.
2. The patient's blood pressure (BP) is reasonably controlled (<160/90 mmHg).

The patient should also have an adequate haemoglobin level (8 g/L) and an US scan to exclude obstruction. Once consent is obtained, the patient is placed supine and an US scanner is used to locate the kidney. It is usually fairly superficial (2–5 cm beneath the skin) and extra-peritoneal, so there is no overlying bowel. Local anaesthetic is applied and a spring-loaded needle inserted into the upper pole (avoiding the vessels and ureter, which are at the lower pole). A single core is usually adequate for diagnosis. Pressure is applied to the site, and the patient placed on bed rest for 6 hours, with frequent monitoring of BP and heart rate. Macroscopic haematuria occurs in <5% and bleeding usually stops spontaneously. Occasionally, radiological embolisation of a bleeding vessel may be required.

Management of post-transplant ATN

It is important to optimise fluid balance to ensure adequate renal perfusion but avoid fluid overload. The latter often necessitates the removal of large amounts of fluid during dialysis, precipitating hypotension and further exacerbating ATN. The recovery from ATN is slowed by the presence of nephrotoxins, such as calcineurin inhibitors (CNIs). Therefore patients are often given reduced doses of CNIs while they have ATN, or in some cases, CNIs are completely withdrawn. Immunosuppression is maintained with oral steroids, mycophenolate and/or induction agents.

Clinical course of post-transplant ATN

The recovery from ATN in transplant kidneys (as in native kidneys) is variable and may take days to weeks, or very occasionally a number of months. Around 5% of patients with DGF never develop graft function. This is termed as primary non-function.

DGF does carry long-term prognostic significance for allografts. In DBD donor kidneys, it is associated with an increased risk of acute rejection and a reduction in long-term graft survival.

(a) Types of rejection

	Hyperacute	Acute T cell-mediated	Acute antibody-mediated	'Chronic' *
Timing	Immediate	1 week – 6 months	1 week – 6 months	Month 1 onwards
Principal immune mediators	Pre-formed antibody, complement	Cytotoxic (CD8) T cells	Antibody, complement, phagocytes	Immune + non-immune mechanisms
Treatment	None (graft nephrectomy)	IV methyl prednisolone increase in maintenance immunosuppression	Plasma exchange, ATG, increase in maintenance immunosuppression	Control BP, minmise exposure to CNIs

* Chronic rejection no longer exists as an entity. The latest Banff classification (2007) distinguishes chronic antibody-mediated rejection and 'tubular atrophy and interstitial fibrosis'

(b) Acute T cell-mediated rejection – immunological mechanisms

1 Antigen presentation – APCs present alloantigen (A) to alloreactive T cells in the context of MHC (signal 1). A co-stimulatory signal is also required (signal 2), provided via the interaction of pairs of costimulatory molecules

2 T cell activation and cytokine production – TCR ligation leads to the dephosphorylation of NFAT, allowing its translocation to the nucleus where it drives the transcription of cytokines (e.g. IL-2). There is also an up-regulation of expression of the α-chain of the IL-2 receptor (CD25), which complexes with the β and γ chains to form a high-affinity receptor

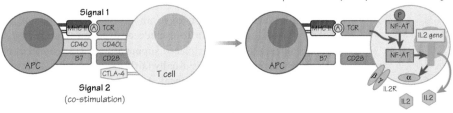

3 Activated CD4 T cells stimulate CD8 T cells via the production of IL-2 – Once activated within an allograft, cytotoxic T cells can damage allograft cells. CD4 T cells also produce cytokines which activate phagocytes, e.g. IFN-γ. These lymphocytes and phagocytes can be observed infiltrating the interstitium, tubules (tubulitis) and vessels (arteritis)

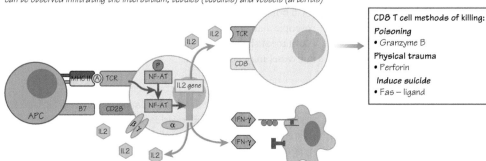

CD8 T cell methods of killing:

Poisoning
• Granzyme B

Physical trauma
• Perforin

Induce suicide
• Fas – ligand

Biopsy findings

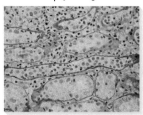

Infiltration of mononuclear cells into tubular walls (tubulitis)

Banff classification of TMR

IA Significant interstitial infiltrate (>25% parenchyma) + moderate tubulitis
IB Significant interstitial infiltrate (>25% parenchyma) + severe tubulitis
IIA Mild-moderate intimal arteritis
IIB Severe intimal arteritis
III Transluminal arteritis + fibrinoid necrosis

(c) Acute antibody-mediated rejection – immunological mechanisms

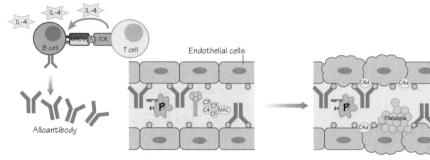

1 Alloreactive B cells produce donor-specific antibody (with T cell help). This antibody binds to endothelial cells within the allograft

2 Deposited antibody activates phagocytes ((P) via Fc receptors) and complement (via the classical pathway)

3 Complement activation leads to C4d deposition. The damage to endothelium results in platelet activation and aggregation. This may be severe enough to completely occlude the lumen of the vessel

Biopsy findings

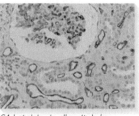

C4d staining in all peritubular capillaries

Banff classification of AMR
C4d+, circulating DSA+
I ATN-like minimal inflammation
II Capillary and glomerular inflammation (neutrophils) or thrombosis
III Transluminal arteritis + fibrinoid necrosis

Transplantation at a Glance, First Edition. Menna Clatworthy, Christopher Watson, Michael Allison and John Dark.

Immunologically mediated allograft damage or rejection may be hyperacute, acute or chronic. Acute rejection is classified as acute cellular/T cell-mediated rejection or acute antibody-mediated/humoral rejection, according to which arm of the immune system is principally involved in mediating allograft damage.

Hyperacute rejection

Hyperacute rejection occurs immediately post-transplant (within minutes to hours) in recipients who have pre-formed, complement-fixing donor-specific antibodies (DSA, typically ABO or HLA). On perfusion of the transplant with the recipient's blood, these antibodies bind to endothelial cells activating complement and phagocytes. This results in endothelial damage, platelet aggregation and rapid arterial and venous thrombosis with subsequent allograft infarction. Once initiated, the process is essentially untreatable, and inevitably leads to allograft loss. Historically, the first attempts at transplantation were performed across blood groups, leading to hyperacute rejection and rapid graft loss. In the current era, hyperacute rejection is very rare, and usually only occurs if there is a mistake in performing the cross-match or transcribing a blood group.

Acute cellular rejection

The most common type of rejection is acute cellular rejection (also known as T cell-mediated rejection [TMR]), occurring in 20–25% of transplants, usually within the first 6 months post-transplant. Patients present with unexplained deterioration in transplant function should undergo an ultrasound scan to exclude obstruction, a urine dipstick and culture to exclude infection, and should have their CNI levels assessed to exclude toxicity. If no alternative cause for decline in graft function is identified, a transplant biopsy is performed.

Immunological mechanisms

TMR occurs when there is presentation of donor antigen to recipient CD4 T cells by antigen-presenting cells (APCs), which may be donor- or recipient-derived (direct antigen presentation = donor MHCI/II/APC; indirect antigen presentation = recipient MHC Class II/APC; *see* Chapter 9). Following antigen presentation, and the provision of co-stimulation through the interaction of surface pairs of co-stimulatory molecules, activated CD4 T cells provide help to CD8 (cytotoxic) T cells, phagocytes and B cells, leading to their infiltration into the graft. Cytotoxic T cells damage and destroy target cells via the production of perforin and granzyme, and through the induction of Fas/Fas ligand-mediated apoptosis.

Biopsy findings

Renal allograft pathology is categorised according to the Banff classification. This is a set of guidelines devised by an international consortium of transplant histopathologists who originally met in the Canadian city of Banff. They are regularly updated to incorporate advances in techniques and in the understanding of pathophysiology.

TMR can affect the tubules and interstitium, causing an interstitial lymphocytic infiltrate and tubulitis (Banff 1 TMR) and, in more severe cases, an arteritis (Banff 2 TMR).

Treatment

The treatment for TMR is high-dose steroid (e.g. 0.5–1 g boluses of methyl prednisolone on three successive days). Baseline maintenance immunosuppression is also increased to prevent recurrent rejection. Most (80–90%) episodes of acute cellular are amenable to treatment with corticosteroids. If the patient's creatinine does not fall in response to corticosteroids (steroid-resistant TMR) then further treatment with a lymphocyte-depleting agent such as anti-thymocyte globulin (ATG) is undertaken. ATG causes profound lymphopaenia, therefore maintenance doses of anti-proliferative agents (azathioprine or mycophenolate) should be omitted during the 10–14 days of ATG administration.

Acute antibody-mediated rejection

Acute antibody-mediated rejection (AMR) occurs in around 2–4% of transplants. The diagnosis requires:
- a decline in allograft function
- the presence of donor-specific HLA antibodies
- the presence of C4d in peritubular capillaries (PTC) on biopsy
- the presence of acute tissue injury (e.g. capillaritis) on biopsy.

Recent studies suggest that non-HLA antibodies, including those recognising major histocompatibility complex class I-related chain A and B antigens (MICA and MICB) and angiotensin II type I receptor may also have an adverse impact on allograft outcomes.

Immunological mechanisms

DSA are produced by terminally differentiated B cells, either short-lived plasmablasts or long-lived bone marrow plasma cells. These antibodies bind to endothelium and activate complement via the classical pathway. Deposited antibody will also activate phagocytes with Fc receptors, including neutrophils.

Biopsy findings

C4d (a degradation product of C4) can be identified on peritubular capillaries and may be focal (<50% of PTCs) or diffuse (>50% of PTCs). Peritubulary capillaries may also contain inflammatory cells (capillaritis) or there may be a more severe arteritis.

There is an increasing, but unresolved, debate about whether peritubular C4d staining in the absence of graft dysfunction has prognostic significance and warrants treatment.

Treatment

AMR is treated by removing DSA via plasma exchange or immunoadsorption, and preventing antibody-associated inflammation with corticosteroids and lymphocyte depletion with ATG. The treatment strategy should also aim to prevent the synthesis of further antibody; however, this is difficult to achieve with current therapies.

In *de novo* AMR in a previously non-sensitised patient, some DSA may be produced by short-lived splenic plasmablasts. These may be reduced by treatment with the CD20 antibody rituximab, as some of these plasmablasts continue to express CD20, and their B cell precursors will also be depleted. In sensitised patients, long-lived bone marrow plasma cells may be the source of antibody, replenished by memory B cells. These are not amenable to rituximab treatment but DSA-producing plasma cells may be sensitive to proteosome inhibition with bortezomib.

An alternative to antibody elimination is to block antibody-mediated graft injury. Eculizumab, an antibody against the C5 complement component, is effective in preventing complement-mediated red cell lysis in patients with paroxysmal nocturnal haemoglobinuria. Recent data suggest that eculizumab may also be effective in preventing DSA-mediated complement activation in the allograft. Even with treatment, AMR may result in chronic allograft damage and is a much more serious condition than TMR.

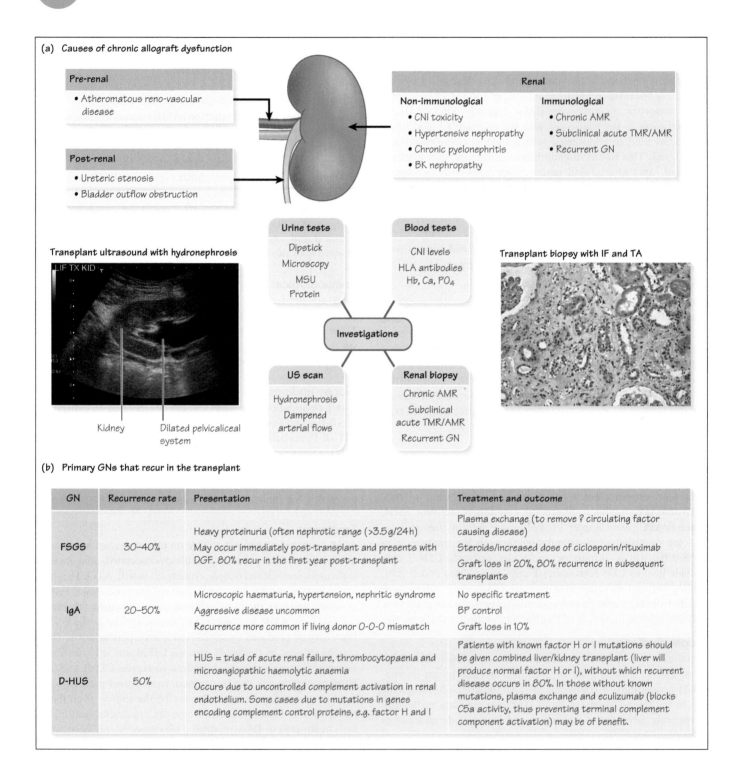

(a) Causes of chronic allograft dysfunction

Pre-renal
- Atheromatous reno-vascular disease

Post-renal
- Ureteric stenosis
- Bladder outflow obstruction

Renal

Non-immunological
- CNI toxicity
- Hypertensive nephropathy
- Chronic pyelonephritis
- BK nephropathy

Immunological
- Chronic AMR
- Subclinical acute TMR/AMR
- Recurrent GN

Transplant ultrasound with hydronephrosis

LIF TX KID

Kidney — Dilated pelvicaliceal system

Urine tests
Dipstick
Microscopy
MSU
Protein

Blood tests
CNI levels
HLA antibodies
Hb, Ca, PO_4

Investigations

US scan
Hydronephrosis
Dampened arterial flows

Renal biopsy
Chronic AMR
Subclinical acute TMR/AMR
Recurrent GN

Transplant biopsy with IF and TA

(b) Primary GNs that recur in the transplant

GN	Recurrence rate	Presentation	Treatment and outcome
FSGS	30–40%	Heavy proteinuria (often nephrotic range (>3.5 g/24 h)) May occur immediately post-transplant and presents with DGF. 80% recur in the first year post-transplant	Plasma exchange (to remove ? circulating factor causing disease) Steroids/increased dose of ciclosporin/rituximab Graft loss in 20%, 80% recurrence in subsequent transplants
IgA	20–50%	Microscopic haematuria, hypertension, nephritic syndrome Aggressive disease uncommon Recurrence more common if living donor 0-0-0 mismatch	No specific treatment BP control Graft loss in 10%
D-HUS	50%	HUS = triad of acute renal failure, thrombocytopaenia and microangiopathic haemolytic anaemia Occurs due to uncontrolled complement activation in renal endothelium. Some cases due to mutations in genes encoding complement control proteins, e.g. factor H and I	Patients with known factor H or I mutations should be given combined liver/kidney transplant (liver will produce normal factor H or I), without which recurrent disease occurs in 80%. In those without known mutations, plasma exchange and eculizumab (blocks C5a activity, thus preventing terminal complement component activation) may be of benefit.

Chronic, progressive loss of allograft function beginning months or years after transplant may have a number of causes, both immunological and non-immunological. Previously, the terms chronic rejection or chronic allograft nephropathy were used to describe this gradual attrition of graft function. However, the most recent Banff classification advises distinguishing chronic antibody-mediated rejection (as evidenced by vascular changes and persistent C4d staining on biopsy in the presence of donor-specific antibodies [DSA]) from interstitial fibrosis and tubular atrophy (which can be caused by a number of factors, including chronic hypertension and CNI).

Transplantation at a Glance, First Edition. Menna Clatworthy, Christopher Watson, Michael Allison and John Dark.

Non-immunological chronic allograft dysfunction

Causes

1 Pre-renal causes:
   (a) atheromatous vascular disease
   (b) hypertension (in donor and/or recipient).
2 Renal causes:
   (a) Calcineurin inhibitor (CNI) toxicity
   (b) BK virus nephropathy
   (c) recurrent pyelonephritis
   (d) diabetic nephropathy.
3 Post-renal:
   (a) ureteric obstruction
   (b) bladder outflow obstruction.

Many of these factors are modifiable (e.g. recipient hypertension, CNI toxicity), therefore it is important to identify them as early as possible by taking a careful history and performing a detailed examination.

History and examination

A history of recurrent urinary tract infections (UTIs) and other urological symptoms should be sought; medications should be reviewed, with particular attention given to CNI dose, and to nephrotoxins such as non-steroidal anti-inflammatory drugs (NSAIDs). A history of smoking and diabetes together with the presence of arterial/transplant bruits, raises the possibility of atheromatous disease affecting the graft. Current blood pressure (BP) should be assessed, as well as a review of previous BP. Patients with chronic urinary obstruction may have a palpable bladder.

Investigations

Blood tests
- Sequential serum creatinine measurement (to estimate rate of decline in renal function).
- CNI levels (current and historical).
- HLA antibody screen (the presence of DSA would suggest an immunological cause of graft dysfunction).

Urine tests
- Urine dipstick/analysis – proteinuria/albumin–creatinine ratio (ACR) or protein-creatinine ratio (PCR).
- Urine cytology – decoy cells in BK nephropathy.
- Mid-steam urine (MSU).

Radiological investigations
- Ultrasound (US): hydronephrosis indicative of obstruction; dampened Doppler flow suggestive of transplant renal artery stenosis.
- MAG3 – a mercaptoacetyltriglycine radionuclide scan to confirm obstruction if US suspicious.
- Renal transplant angiogram – if arterial stenosis suspected.

Renal biopsy
If the above investigations do not reveal an obvious cause for the decline in graft function, then the patient should proceed to a transplant biopsy to exclude an immunological cause of graft dysfunction such as chronic antibody-mediated rejection (AMR) and recurrent glomerulonephritis (GN).

Commonly observed chronic histological changes include interstitial fibrosis (IF) and tubular atrophy (TA), which are graded according to the amount of cortical area involved:

Grade	Cortical involvement
I (mild)	<25% of cortical area
II (moderate)	25–50% of cortical area
III (severe)	>50% of cortical area

In addition to IF/TA, there is frequently vascular damage, with intimal thickening and glomerulosclerosis. More specific features of CNI toxicity include tubular cell vacuolation, arteriolar hyalinosis and thrombotic microangiopathy.

Management

This depends on the cause. Arterial stenoses should be treated with angioplasty where possible; ureteric obstruction resolved via stent insertion and surgical intervention; and bladder outflow obstruction treated via catheter insertion and/or treatment of prostatic disease. More general measures include tight blood pressure control (<130/80 mmHg), treatment of proteinuria with ACEi/ARB, and treatment of chronic kidney disease-associated anaemia and bone-mineral disease. Where CNI toxicity is suspected, CNIs may be minimised or even withdrawn, with conversion to sirolimus (which is non-nephrotoxic).

Immunological chronic allograft dysfunction

Causes

1 Chronic AMR
2 Subclinical acute TMR or AMR
3 Recurrent GN

History, examination, and investigation

Recurrent disease
- Review the cause of renal failure; is it a GN known to recur in transplants (e.g. focal segmental glomerulosclerosis [FSGS], IgA)?

Rejection
- Have there been episodes of acute rejection previously, particularly steroid-resistant rejection or AMR?
- Compliance to immunosuppression should be assessed, both by direct questioning and by reviewing longitudinal CNI levels.
- The presence of current or previous DSA increases the likelihood of chronic AMR, as does a high degree of HLA mismatch.

Diagnosis ultimately requires a renal transplant biopsy. Chronic AMR is evidenced by diffuse peritubular capillary (PTC) C4d staining, transplant glomerulopathy (double contouring in peripheral capillary loops) and PTC basement membrane multi-layering.

Management

Chronic AMR has no proven treatment. Switching immunosuppression to include tacrolimus and mycophenolate may be helpful. Rituximab is also being trialled in patients with chronic AMR but the prognosis remains poor, with 50% loss of graft within 5 years.

Subclinical TMR and AMR should be treated as described in Chapter 23.

Recurrent GNs are seldom amenable to treatment, with the exception of FSGS or atypical/diarrhoea-negative haemolytic uraemic syndrome (D-HUS), which can be treated with plasma exchange or eculizumab (atypical HUS).

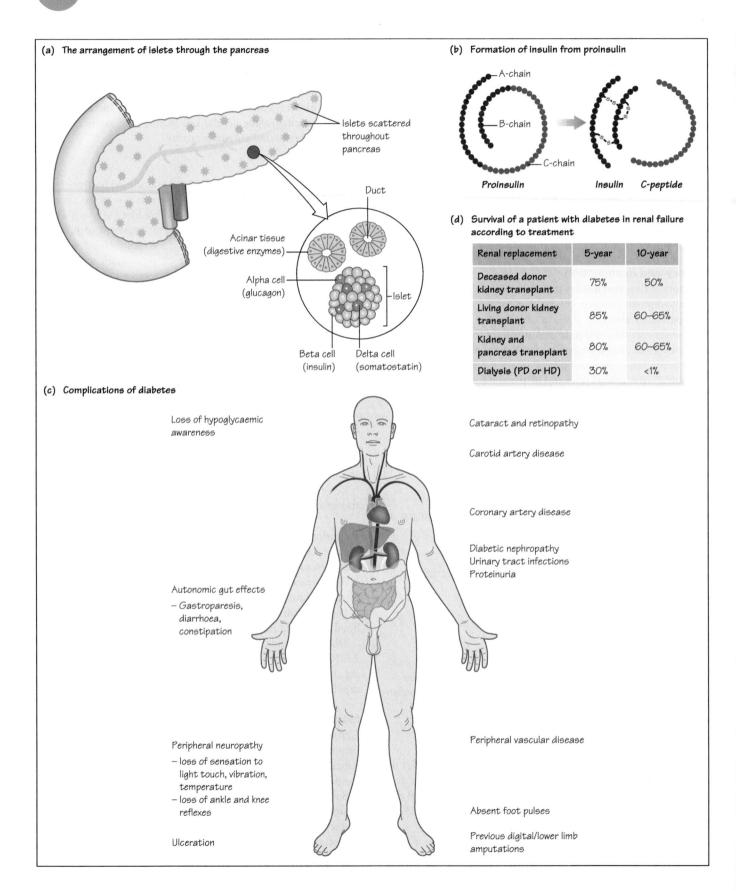

(a) The arrangement of islets through the pancreas

Islets scattered throughout pancreas

Duct

Acinar tissue (digestive enzymes)

Alpha cell (glucagon)

Islet

Beta cell (insulin)

Delta cell (somatostatin)

(b) Formation of insulin from proinsulin

A-chain

B-chain

C-chain

Proinsulin

Insulin

C-peptide

(d) Survival of a patient with diabetes in renal failure according to treatment

Renal replacement	5-year	10-year
Deceased donor kidney transplant	75%	50%
Living donor kidney transplant	85%	60–65%
Kidney and pancreas transplant	80%	60–65%
Dialysis (PD or HD)	30%	<1%

(c) Complications of diabetes

Loss of hypoglycaemic awareness

Autonomic gut effects
– Gastroparesis, diarrhoea, constipation

Peripheral neuropathy
– loss of sensation to light touch, vibration, temperature
– loss of ankle and knee reflexes

Ulceration

Cataract and retinopathy

Carotid artery disease

Coronary artery disease

Diabetic nephropathy
Urinary tract infections
Proteinuria

Peripheral vascular disease

Absent foot pulses

Previous digital/lower limb amputations

Transplantation at a Glance, First Edition. Menna Clatworthy, Christopher Watson, Michael Allison and John Dark.

66 © 2012 John Wiley & Sons, Ltd. Published 2012 by John Wiley & Sons, Ltd.

Diabetes mellitus

Diabetes mellitus is characterised by high blood sugars due to insufficient insulin or insensitivity to the actions of insulin.

Type 1 diabetes is due to an autoimmune destruction of the insulin-producing beta cells. Patients typically present in childhood or adolescence with ketoacidosis and are insulin-dependent from the outset. Autoantibodies to islet cell antigens are frequently detectable.

Type 2 diabetes is the result of insulin resistance, and typically occurs in older and more obese patients. They are usually non-ketotic at presentation and do not immediately require insulin. Initially the beta cells attempt to compensate for the insulin resistance by increasing production; however, with time, the beta cells burn out.

Other forms of diabetes: *Gestational diabetes (GDM)* – occurs in pregnancy, has similar features to type 2 diabetes and often resolves after delivery. Many patients with GDM will go on to develop type 2 diabetes later in life.

Maturity onset diabetes of the young (MODY) – caused by single gene mutations (e.g. HNF-1α gene) that result in abnormal beta cell function, insulin processing or insulin action.

Pancreatic pathology – pancreatitis, pancreatic cancer, cystic fibrosis, haemochromatosis and pancreatectomy may all cause diabetes.

Insulin production

Around 1% of the cells in the pancreas are within the islets of Langerhans; these are small clusters of hormone-secreting cells that are scattered throughout the pancreas. One of these hormone-secreting cell types is the beta cell, which secretes insulin in response to high blood glucose. The islets also contain other hormone-secreting cells, such as alpha cells producing glucagon, and delta cells producing somatostatin.

Within the beta cells insulin is produced as a precursor called proinsulin, a single polypeptide chain which folds such that the two ends of the chain become bound by two pairs of disulphide bonds. This polypeptide is then cleaved into three fragments, the A, B and C peptides. A and B form the insulin molecule, and the C peptide is released. Measurement of C peptide in the serum can be used to determine whether a potential recipient makes their own insulin (i.e. not type 1), since artificial insulin does not contain this peptide.

High concentrations of glucose entering the beta cells trigger release of insulin. This insulin is secreted directly into the portal circulation to have its initial effect on the liver, where it is required to permit entry of glucose into the cells.

The complications of diabetes

The main complication of diabetes is the development of accelerated vascular disease. This is particularly marked in patients with poor glucose control and those who smoke. Vascular complications are categorised according to the size of vessels involved:

Macrovascular complications

1 Coronary artery disease: angina and/or myocardial infarction.
2 Peripheral vascular disease (PVD) characterised by claudication, rest pain, ulceration and gangrene.
3 Cerebrovascular disease, manifesting with transient ischaemic attacks (TIA), amaurosis fugax or cerebrovascular accident.

Microvascular complications

Retinopathy Microvascular disease affecting the retinal vessels is classified according to severity and whether the macula is involved.
• *Background* – microaneurysms (dots) and microhaemorrhages (blots), hard exudates.
• *Pre-proliferative* – cotton wool spots (soft exudates indicative of retinal infarcts), more extensive microhaemorrhage.
• *Proliferative* – new vessel formation.
• *Maculopathy* – changes described in background or pre-proliferative retinopathy affecting the macula.
If there is significant haemorrhage then retinal detachment may occur. Diabetes is also associated with cataract formation.

Neuropathy A number of types of diabetic neuropathy occur.

Peripheral sensory neuropathy – typically in a 'glove and stocking' distribution. Vibration sensation is lost early. In advanced disease, sensation in the feet may be completely absent, resulting in unnoticed trauma and subsequent ulceration. In the presence of PVD, the blood supply is impaired, leading to poor healing, sometimes necessitating amputation.

Autonomic neuropathy – symptoms vary and include gustatory sweating, gastroparesis (vomiting and nausea), bladder dysfunction, erectile dysfunction and postural hypotension (due to loss of regulation of vascular tone). Of most significance is the loss of awareness of hypoglycaemia. Hypoglycaemia is normally accompanied by tremor, sweating and palpitations due to the release of adrenaline (epinephrine) in response to low brain glucose (neuroglycopaenia). This has the additional role of stimulating glycogenolysis and gluconeogenesis in the liver. This compensatory adrenaline release is lost in patients with hypoglycaemic unawareness. The net result is that blood sugar may fall dangerously low, causing significant brain damage or death.

Painful neuropathy – damage to sensory nerves may lead to a burning pain or sensitivity to touch.

Mononeuritis multiplex – may affect any peripheral nerve.

Diabetic amyotrophy – painful wasting and weakness of quadriceps.

Nephropathy Patients with type 1 diabetes frequently develop renal involvement. At least 25% of diabetics diagnosed before the age of 25 years will go onto to develop end-stage renal failure.

Diabetic nephropathy is characterised by albuminuria, which may progress to heavy proteinuria with decline in glomerular filtration rate (GFR). Histologically, there is basement membrane thickening and glomerulosclerosis, which may be diffuse or nodular (Kimmelstiel–Wilson lesions). Diabetic patients are also more susceptible to urinary tract infections, which may contribute to chronic renal damage.

In the UK, diabetes is the most common cause of ESRF requiring renal replacement therapy. Diabetics on dialysis have a very poor outlook, with a 30% 5-year survival.

Indications

Both pancreas and islet transplantation are for the treatment of diabetes mellitus. Since both require standard immunosuppression, the benefits of the procedure have to outweigh the risks, and the side effects and complications of immunosuppression. Therefore it is generally agreed that the patient should have a life-threatening complication of diabetes, such as hypoglycaemic unawareness, or that they require immunosuppression for another reason, such as a kidney transplant.

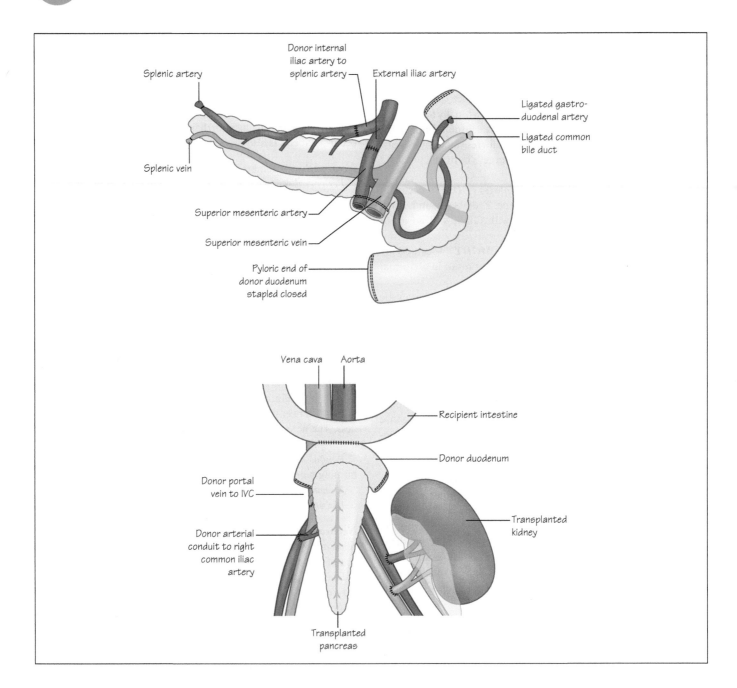

Splenic artery

Donor internal iliac artery to splenic artery

External iliac artery

Ligated gastro-duodenal artery

Ligated common bile duct

Splenic vein

Superior mesenteric artery

Superior mesenteric vein

Pyloric end of donor duodenum stapled closed

Vena cava

Aorta

Recipient intestine

Donor duodenum

Donor portal vein to IVC

Donor arterial conduit to right common iliac artery

Transplanted kidney

Transplanted pancreas

Categories of transplant

Simultaneous pancreas and kidney (SPK, 80%)

The pancreas is transplanted at the same time as a kidney from the same deceased donor. The recipient is in kidney failure, and either on or within a few months of starting dialysis. This combination is a bigger surgical operation, but has the benefit that the kidney can be used as a surrogate to monitor rejection of both grafts.

Pancreas after kidney transplantation (PAK, 15%)

Where patients have previously undergone a kidney transplant, e.g. from a live donor, or an SPK where the pancreas has failed, a subsequent solitary pancreas can be performed. This may affect the residual renal function, which needs to be carefully assessed.

Pancreas transplant alone (PTA, 5%)

Indicated for life-threatening hypoglycaemic unawareness.

Transplantation at a Glance, First Edition. Menna Clatworthy, Christopher Watson, Michael Allison and John Dark.

Patient assessment

Pancreas transplantation is a major surgical operation with a higher than average risk of complications that might necessitate further surgery. Candidates for the procedure are carefully assessed with this in mind.

The basic clinical assessment of a potential pancreas recipient is similar to that of a potential kidney transplant recipient. Particular note is taken of active ulceration or sepsis, which is a contraindication to transplantation. Examination should assess the degree of neuropathy, in addition to a full cardiovascular, respiratory and abdominal examination.

A thorough cardiovascular assessment is essential, and comprises ECG and echocardiography, with stress imaging (dobutamine stress echo or radionuclide scan); coronary angiography, carotid duplex scanning and abdominal duplex or CT are frequently required. In addition, screening for gallstones is worthwhile since cholecystectomy at the time of transplant may avoid cholecystitis in the post-operative period.

Transplantation

The donor organ

The pancreas is transplanted as a bloc of tissue, which also includes the donor duodenum. The pancreatic arterial supply comes from the splenic artery and inferior pancreaticoduodenal branch of the superior mesenteric artery; these two arteries are joined together on the back table before surgery utilising the donor's common iliac artery bifurcation as a conduit, giving just one arterial anastomosis in the recipient. The venous drainage is via a 1 cm stump of donor portal vein.

Exocrine drainage

The pancreas produces around 1.5 litres of enzyme-rich secretions each day. This must be drained either by anastomosing the donor duodenum to the dome of the bladder (bladder drainage) or to a segment or Roux-en-Y loop of small bowel (enteric drainage). Bladder drainage has the advantage that the urinary amylase concentration will give an indication of the function of the graft; it has the disadvantage of massive bicarbonate loss and may cause a chemical cystitis necessitating subsequent conversion to enteric drainage. Most centres now perform primary enteric drainage, although bladder drainage may be preferred for solitary transplants where the ability to monitor the urinary amylase may be more important.

Venous drainage

The venous drainage may either be fashioned by anastomosing the donor portal vein to the inferior vena cava (IVC) or one of its tributaries, or to the superior mesenteric vein (SMV). The IVC has the advantage of being simple; the SMV is more physiological, because insulin is delivered to the portal circulation.

Systemic venous drainage (i.e. to the IVC) results in higher systemic insulin levels and a delayed response to increasing glucose and decreasing glucose, the latter accounting for hypoglycaemic episodes that these patients sometimes experience.

The pancreas is usually placed intraperitoneal through a midline incision, although extraperitoneal placement like a kidney is possible so long as a window into the peritoneum is made to facilitate drainage of the inflammatory exudate that arises following transplantation.

Immunosuppression and prophylaxis

Lymphocyte-depleting monoclonal antibodies such as alemtuzumab are used to permit steroid-free immunosuppression; tacrolimus and mycophenolate are the usual maintenance agents. Care should be taken with sirolimus because its ability to delay healing may have catastrophic consequences should foot ulceration occur.

In addition to the usual prophylaxis given for kidney transplantation, prophylactic antifungal (e.g. fluconazole) and broad-spectrum antimicrobial (e.g. meropenem) agents are given because the duodenal contents may be contaminated.

Complications

Surgical complications

Thrombosis occurs in 5–10% of pancreas transplants. There are several reasons.

• The splenic and superior mesenteric arteries and portal vein are large vessels capable of handling flows of 1.5 L/min; in isolation the pancreas has a blood supply nearer 100 ml/min so there is significant stasis in the vessels.

• Pancreatitis occurs secondary to ischaemic damage. This also predisposes to thrombosis.

• Diabetes is often associated with a hypercoagulable state.

Bleeding. The mesenteric vessels pass through the neck of the pancreas and are oversewn along the cut edge of the mesentry; the vessels to the spleen and inferior mesenteric vein (IMV) are also ligated. Nevertheless, bleeding on reperfusion and post-operatively is common, and frequently requires a second laparotomy. The necessity to give antithrombotic prophylaxis increases the risk of bleeding.

Intra-abdominal hypertension requiring interposition mesh closure of the abdominal wall may result from the extra volume of tissue transplanted into often small abdomens.

General complications

As with any abdominal surgery there is a risk of chest infection, wound infection and wound breakdown. Patients are also at risk of the long- and short-term complications of immunosuppression.

Foot ulceration, particularly heel ulceration following prolonged immobilisation, is a risk so patients are nursed on an air mattress to minimise pressure.

Metabolic complications include bicarbonate loss from a bladder-drained pancreas and hypoglycaemia from a systemic venous-drained pancreas.

Long-term outcomes

Patients are generally insulin independent from the time of transplantation. The 1-year graft and patient survival are 90% and 98%; thereafter the half-life of a pancreas transplant is around 10 years if transplanted with a kidney, and less if transplanted in isolation (PAK, PTA). Pancreas transplantation has a higher 1-year mortality than kidney transplantation alone, but a far superior 10-year survival due largely to beneficial effects in reducing cardiac events.

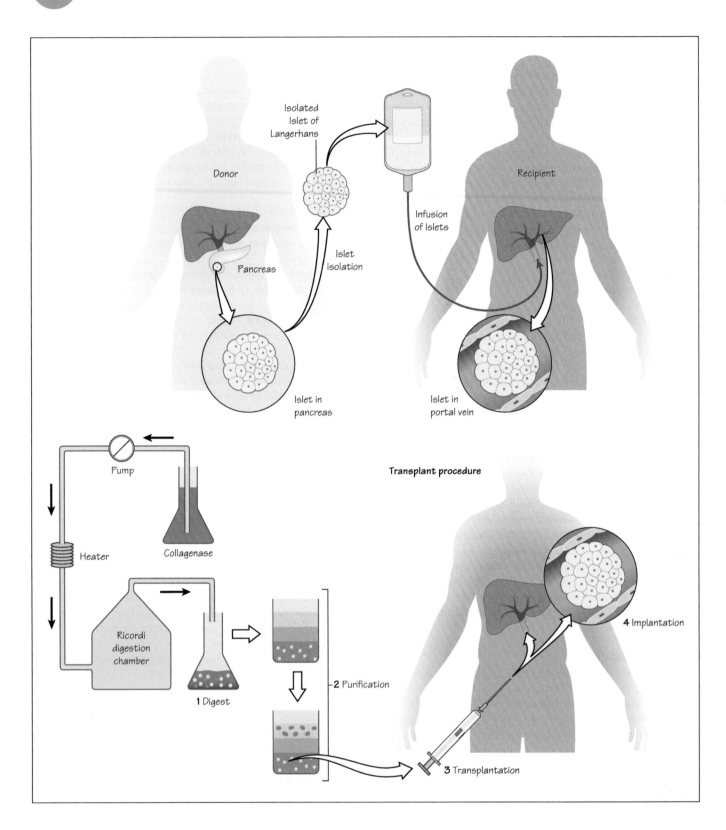

Indications for islet transplantation

1 *Islet transplantation alone* (ITA) is indicated for life-threatening hypoglycaemic unawareness.

2 *Islet after kidney transplantation* (IAK), where patients are already taking immunosuppression and have life-threatening complications of their diabetes.

3 *Autologous islet transplantation* in patients with chronic pancreatitis undergoing pancreatectomy. Their pancreas is processed, the islets extracted and then infused into their liver.

Assessment for transplantation

Optimisation of insulin therapy is the first part of the assessment to see whether diabetic management can be improved without transplantation. This may involve more frequent insulin injections or a trial of insulin-pump therapy.

The assessment of fitness for the transplant procedure is similar to that required for whole pancreas transplantation, except that the patient does not need to be as cardiovascularly robust. Nevertheless, major cardiac disease is still a contraindication if it precludes long-term patient survival.

Islet isolation and transplantation

Purification and transplantation

Islet transplantation has been the goal of research ever since Banting and Best proved that it was the islets that produced insulin. However, the islets are scattered throughout the pancreas so the process of separating them from the acinar pancreatic tissue (which makes the digestive enzymes) has proved a formidable challenge.

The current process involves separate stages.

1 *Digestion.* The enzyme collagenase is injected into the pancreatic duct to break down the collagen holding the islets in place. This takes place in a chamber at 37°C.

2 *Blocking of digestion.* As the islets break free they pass out of the digestion chamber into another container where the enzyme digestion is stopped by cooling to 4°C.

3 *Purification.* The islet tissue, together with a lot of pancreatic acinar tissue, is centrifuged over density gradients to isolate the islets.

4 *Transplantation.* Purified islets are then injected via a needle inserted through the skin, through the liver and into the portal vein, where they embolise into the smaller venous tributaries.

The whole process is rather wasteful of islets; typically only a half of the 1 million islets in a pancreas finish up as purified, transplantable islets; the remainder fragment into smaller clusters of cells due to too much exposure to collagenase, or remain adherent to the gland due to too little exposure.

Following transplantation only around a half of the transplanted islets successfully implant into the liver and produce insulin. Typically more than 5000 islet equivalents are required to be transplanted per kilogram weight of the recipient.

Immunosuppression

Patients receive similar immunosuppression to kidney transplant recipients, with the exception of avoiding steroids. The current immunosuppressants do not facilitate successful transplantation.

* Calcineurin inhibitors such as tacrolimus are islet toxic.
* Sirolimus appears to reduce engraftment, possibly via inhibition of vascular endothelial growth factor.

* Mycophenolate and azathioprine are insufficient to prevent rejection.

Complications

Procedural complications

* *Abnormalities of liver biochemistry.*
* *Bleeding from the punctured liver* is common (15%), and may occasionally require blood transfusion. It often presents with abdominal and right shoulder tip pain. The risk is reduced by injection of sealant along the track (e.g. fibrin glue), although that increases the risk of thrombosis.
* *Portal vein thrombosis* (4%) arising as a complication of embolisation. Diabetic patients are often procoagulant and thrombosis is a risk.
* *Biliary leak,* resulting in abdominal pain.
* *Gall bladder puncture,* resulting in biliary leak; other inadvertent organ puncture is also possible.
* *Fatty liver* (hepatic steatosis) occurs in the long term, usually focally along portal tracts where islets are functional. These appearances may return to normal after the graft fails.
* *Portal hypertension* may occur with repeated islet infusions. As the islets embolise into the portal vein they progressively block more and more tributaries.

Complications of transplantation

* *Immunosuppression.* Islet transplantation requires equivalent levels of immunosuppression to those needed in kidney transplantation, with the associated drug specific side effects (especially nephrotoxicity) and the adverse consequences of immunosuppression including infection and malignancy.
* *Sensitisation to HLA antigens on the donor,* occurring as part of the rejection process, reduces the pool of donors suitable for subsequent transplants (islets or other organs, e.g. the kidney).

Islet graft failure

Islet graft failure is common, with a 5-year graft survival of around 12%. Although the patient may have returned to insulin, there is often useful insulin production still occurring (as evidenced by the presence of C-peptide in the serum). This is frequently sufficient to stabilise diabetic management and prevent life-threatening hypoglycaemia.

The cause of graft failure is often unclear. There is no way to monitor for rejection, which probably accounts for a significant proportion of graft failures. The innate immune system is very active in the liver and probably accounts for other graft losses, and the concept of 'islet exhaustion' is also proposed to explain poor long term outcomes.

Pancreas or islets?

The results of pancreas transplantation are superior to those of islet transplantation; grafts function better (insulin independence is common) and last longer. However, pancreas transplantation is a large surgical undertaking with significant morbidity and mortality. Islet transplantation is a minor procedure with few complications, but with disappointing long-term results.

At present it is difficult to justify equal access to pancreases for whole organ and islet transplantation, so islet transplantation will remain a secondary procedure.

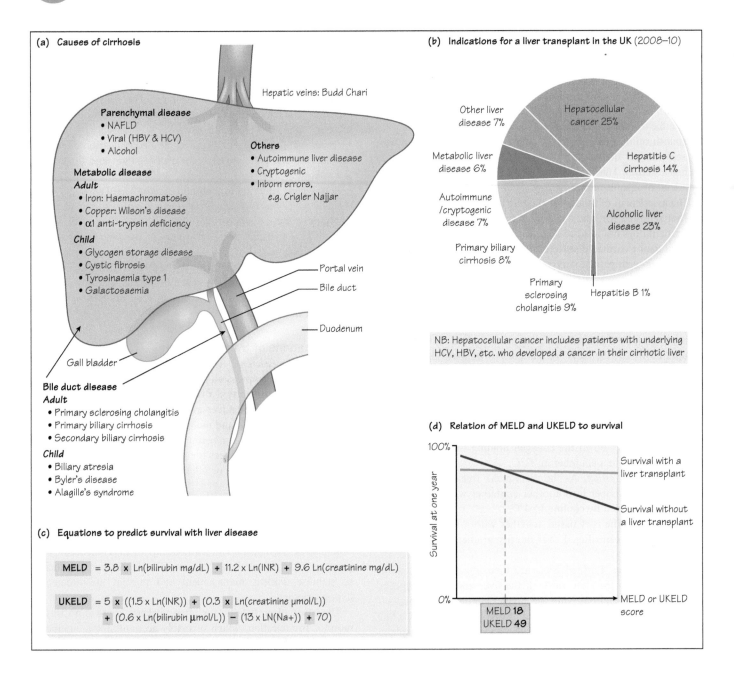

(a) Causes of cirrhosis

Hepatic veins: Budd Chari

Parenchymal disease
- NAFLD
- Viral (HBV & HCV)
- Alcohol

Metabolic disease
Adult
- Iron: Haemachromatosis
- Copper: Wilson's disease
- α1 anti-trypsin deficiency

Child
- Glycogen storage disease
- Cystic fibrosis
- Tyrosinaemia type 1
- Galactosaemia

Others
- Autoimmune liver disease
- Cryptogenic
- Inborn errors, e.g. Crigler Najjar

Portal vein
Bile duct
Duodenum

Gall bladder

Bile duct disease
Adult
- Primary sclerosing cholangitis
- Primary biliary cirrhosis
- Secondary biliary cirrhosis

Child
- Biliary atresia
- Byler's disease
- Alagille's syndrome

(b) Indications for a liver transplant in the UK (2008–10)

- Hepatocellular cancer 25%
- Hepatitis C cirrhosis 14%
- Alcoholic liver disease 23%
- Hepatitis B 1%
- Primary sclerosing cholangitis 9%
- Primary biliary cirrhosis 8%
- Autoimmune /cryptogenic disease 7%
- Metabolic liver disease 6%
- Other liver disease 7%

NB: Hepatocellular cancer includes patients with underlying HCV, HBV, etc. who developed a cancer in their cirrhotic liver

(c) Equations to predict survival with liver disease

MELD = 3.8 x Ln(bilirubin mg/dL) + 11.2 x Ln(INR) + 9.6 Ln(creatinine mg/dL)

UKELD = 5 x ((1.5 x Ln(INR)) + (0.3 x Ln(creatinine µmol/L))
+ (0.6 x Ln(bilirubin µmol/L)) − (13 x LN(Na+)) + 70)

(d) Relation of MELD and UKELD to survival

Survival at one year (100% to 0%)

- Survival with a liver transplant
- Survival without a liver transplant

MELD 18
UKELD 49

MELD or UKELD score

Causes of liver failure

Currently, approximately 85% of liver transplants in the UK are undertaken in adults, the remainder in children. Most (85%) are for chronic liver disease, with only a few for acute liver failure.

Chronic liver disease

Cirrhosis develops as a result of a (usually chronic) insult to the liver, which causes inflammation and liver cell damage, with resultant scarring and regeneration. The common causes of cirrhosis for which liver transplantation is performed are shown in Figure 33. Cirrhosis has four main consequences.

Hepatocellular failure

Hepatocellular failure manifests in three ways.

1 *Impaired protein synthesis*, best monitored by the prothombin time (or its ratio to an international normal value, the INR) and serum albumin. Progressive liver disease results in prolongation of the prothrombin time and a fall in serum albumin concentration. It also results in malnutrition, which may prejudice recovery from transplantation.

2 *Impaired metabolism of toxins* results in encephalopathy, characterised by confusion, somnolence, a 'flapping' hand tremor and coma.

3 *Impaired bilirubin metabolism* resulting in jaundice.

Transplantation at a Glance, First Edition. Menna Clatworthy, Christopher Watson, Michael Allison and John Dark.

72 © 2012 John Wiley & Sons, Ltd. Published 2012 by John Wiley & Sons, Ltd.

Portal hypertension

Portal hypertension is a consequence of the cirrhotic distortion of the liver's architecture, which impedes the passage of portal venous blood, so raising the pressure in the portal circulation. As portal hypertension develops new collateral channels develop, draining blood from the portal to systemic venous system, along the peritoneal attachments of the liver, the ligamentum teres (the obliterated umbilical vein, which reopens in the presence of portal hypertension) and as varices alongside the gastro-oesophageal junction. The collateral vessels around the liver, as well as the abnormal clotting cascade, account for much of the bleeding associated with transplantation of the liver.

Ascites

Ascites is also consequence of portal hypertension and warrants transplantation if it is resistant to standard treatment with diuretics.

Hepatocellular carcinoma (hepatoma)

The chronic inflammatory processes of different aetiologies that lead to cirrhosis also can result in hepatoma formation, particularly when associated with viral infection such as hepatitis C. Because the liver is cirrhotic, insufficient functioning liver would remain if the liver lobe containing tumour was resected, so transplantation is the principle curative treatment. However, very large tumours, or multiple tumours, are less likely to be curable so access to transplantation is restricted to patients with solitary tumours under 5 cm in diameter or, if multiple, no more than three tumours each no greater than 3 cm in diameter – these criteria may vary from country to country.

Other liver tumours, such as cholangiocarcinoma, hepatoblastoma and metastatic neuroendocrine tumours, are associated with early recurrence and are not suitable indications for transplantation.

Clinical features of liver disease which warrant assessment for transplantation

Five clinical features suggest liver transplantation may be required.
1 Jaundice in the context of end-stage liver disease.
2 Intractable ascites (i.e. resistant to treatment).
3 Recurrent or refractory hepatic encephalopathy.
4 Breathlessness due to hepatopulmonary syndrome.
5 Intractable pruritis.

Who to list?

Since donor livers are in short supply it is usual not to offer a transplant to someone whose anticipated life expectancy after a liver transplant is short, and in the UK patients would be expected to have a 50% chance of surviving 5 years following liver transplantation.

When to list?

Assimilating biochemical data can indicate when a patient with chronic liver disease is at a point when transplantation is necessary, that is when their risk of death without a transplant is greater than that with a transplant; to this end a number of predictive equations based on serum bilirubin, INR and renal function have been developed, such as the Model for End-stage Liver Disease (MELD) and the equivalent UK model (UKELD) (*see* Figure 33). A MELD over 18, or UKELD ≥ 49 are taken as indications for transplantation, since at this point the survival following liver transplantation exceeds that without transplantation (9% mortality at 1 year if UKELD = 49).

Acute liver failure

Liver transplantation is indicated as an emergency treatment for patients with unrecoverable acute liver failure. However, the low availability of donor livers means that one in three patients dies while waiting.

Assessing when to list a patient with acute liver failure can be difficult, and reliance is placed on factors that are known to predict poor outcome without transplantation. The Kings College criteria for predicting non-recovery in acute liver failure, and therefore indicating transplantation, are one such example. They are as follows.

Paracetamol poisoning
• Arterial pH <7.3
or
• Grade III or IV encephalopathy *and*
• Prothrombin time >100 s (INR > 6.5) *and*
• Serum creatinine >300 μmol/L

Non-paracetamol acute liver failure
• Prothrombin time >100 s (INR > 6.5) *or* any three of
• Age <10 or >40 years
• Aetiology non-A, non-B; halothane hepatitis; idiosyncratic drug reaction
• Duration of jaundice before encephalopathy >7 days
• Prothrombin time >50 s (INR > 3.5)
• Serum bilirubin >300 μmol/L

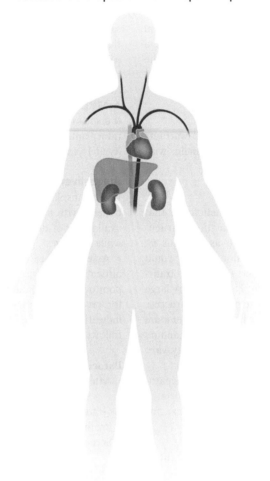

Assessment of the potential liver transplant recipient

Endoscopy
- Oropharynx (smoker/alcoholic)
- Oesophago-gastro-duodenal varices/ulcer/tumours

Cardiac assessment
- Resting ECG
- Echocardiography
- Stress echo/nuclear scan and/or coronary angiography

Liver assessment
- Ultrasound – vessels/tumours
- CT/MR for focal lesions ?tumour
- Staging CT chest if hepatoma

Bone density
- Reduced in presence of cirrhosis

Screening liver blood tests
- Prothrombin time/albumin:
  – synthetic function
- Bilirubin: metabolic dysfunction
- ALT/AST – hepatocellular damage
- ALP – bile duct damage
- Hepatitis viral serology
- Autoimmune serology, e.g. anti-nuclear (ANA), anti-mitochondrial (AMA) and anti-smooth muscle antibodies (SMA)
- Ferritin/iron studies – haemochromatosis
- Serum copper, caeruloplasmin – Wilson's disease
- Alpha 1-antitrypsin level (+ phenotype if low)
- Alphafetoprotein (AFP) – hepatoma marker
- CA19.9 – cholangiocarcinoma tumour marker

Psychiatric assessment
- Particularly important with history of alcohol or drugs and with respect to compliance with post-operative medication

Ophthalmic assessment (slit lamp)
- Kayser–Fleischer rings around iris if Wilson's disease is suspected

Respiratory assessment
- Chest radiograph
- Pulmonary function tests
- Gas transfer
- Arterial blood gases, esp pO_2
- Nuclear medicine shuntogram
- Bubble echocardiography (shunts)

Renal function assessment
- Serum urea and creatinine
- Urinary protein extretion
- Glomerular filtration rate
- Kidney biopsy if renal impairment

Surgical assessment
- Previous upper abdominal surgery
- Presence and location of varices
- Patency of portal vein
- Patency of hepatic artery

Assessment of the transplant candidate

As with renal transplantation, assessment of a potential liver transplant recipient involves not only evaluation of the liver disease for which transplantation is indicated, but also determination of comorbidity that may affect peri- or post-operative morbidity and mortality. Moreover, since liver transplantation is now a successful treatment for liver failure, focus has switched to ensuring long-term survival rather than just surviving the surgical assault. The shortage of organs has necessitated increased selectivity, favouring patients with better anticipated outcomes.

Evaluating the liver disease

Most liver screening tests are repeated to verify the diagnosis and rule out other diseases. These are illustrated in Figure 34.

Liver biopsy may be indicated in patients with a presumed hepatoma but otherwise good function, when biopsy of the background liver will help decide whether a liver resection is possible rather than a transplant. In general, focal lesions are *not* biopsied if they have characteristic radiological features of a hepatoma, due to the risk of seeding the tumour outside the liver.

Upper gastrointestinal endoscopy looking for varices, ulcers and tumours.

Ultrasound examination screens for focal lesions that may represent tumours, and confirms the presence of patent hepatic artery, and portal and hepatic veins. Hepatic vein occlusion suggests Budd Chiari disease.

Further cross-sectional imaging may be required to characterise any focal lesion – hepatomas typically take up contrast in the arterial phase of computed tomography (CT) and 'wash out' leaving a hypodense area in the portal venous phase. Magnetic resonance (MR) imaging may help to define a lesion. The differential diagnosis of small lesions is between regenerative nodule and hepatoma.

Transplantation at a Glance, First Edition. Menna Clatworthy, Christopher Watson, Michael Allison and John Dark.

74 © 2012 John Wiley & Sons, Ltd. Published 2012 by John Wiley & Sons, Ltd.

Nodules that have the typical appearance of tumour are not biopsied for fear of seeding the tumour outside the liver.

Pre-transplant anti-hepatoma therapy, either radiofrequency ablation (RFA) or trans-arterial chemo-embolisation (TACE), are considered as treatment to reduce the growth (and prevent spread) of the tumour while the patient is on the waiting list.

Evaluating the surgical challenge

Previous upper abdominal surgery, particularly procedures in the liver hilum such as cholecystectomy or highly selective vagotomy, result in adhesions, which become very vascular in the presence of portal hypertension and are associated with longer surgery and greater blood loss.

Patency of the portal vein is checked, and if thrombosed, the possibility of performing a graft from the portal vein of the transplant to the superior mesenteric vein or left renal vein of the recipient is assessed. Mesenteric venous thrombosis may be an indication for a multivisceral transplant rather than a liver transplant alone. Portal vein thrombosis in the presence of hepatoma is often due to vascular invasion which precludes liver transplantation.

Hepatic artery anatomy, patency and identification of anomalies is important. If the recipient artery is small or thrombosed, it may be necessary to do a jump graft from the recipient's aorta, so the presence or absence of aortic disease is assessed – it is too late to discover an aortic aneurysm once the liver has been removed.

Evaluating comorbidity

Cardiovascular disease can be difficult to assess. Most liver failure patients have limited exercise tolerance and their vasodilated state, a consequence of liver failure, tends to offload the heart, so masking possible cardiac disease. Echocardiography and stress testing are performed where concern exists.

Portopulmonary hypertension (pressure >25 mmHg) may be suggested on echocardiography. If so, it is confirmed by direct measurement. Severe portopulmonary hypertension (mean pulmonary arterial pressure [MPAP] >50 mmHg) constitutes a contraindication to liver transplantation,

Diabetes is common in patients with chronic liver disease, particularly hepatitis C and non-alcoholic fatty liver disease (NAFLD), and may contribute to cardiovascular disease.

Chronic renal disease has a significant impact on outcome and requires careful assessment. Combined liver and kidney transplant may be preferred in carefully selected patients to improve post-operative outcome.

Respiratory assessment with pulmonary function testing and blood gas analysis is necessary to evaluate any associated lung disease – smoking and alcohol are common bedfellows. Hypoxic patients with hepatopulmonary syndrome due to arteriovenous shunting through the lungs require careful study – high levels of shunting preclude transplantation because adequate oxygenation may not be possible post-operatively. An arterial pO_2 <50 mmHg on room air is a contraindication to transplantation.

Oropharyngeal examination is appropriate in patients with a history of alcohol intake and smoking; oropharyngeal (and oesophageal) cancers are common in this group and easily missed.

Psychiatric evaluation is important where substance misuse has occurred (e.g. alcohol-related liver disease or prior intravenous drug misuse), with particular attention paid to ensuring that adequate support services are in place for the patient in the post-operative period. Such support can minimise the chances of return to alcohol consumption or illicit drug use, which can have a negative impact on patient and graft survival post-transplantation.

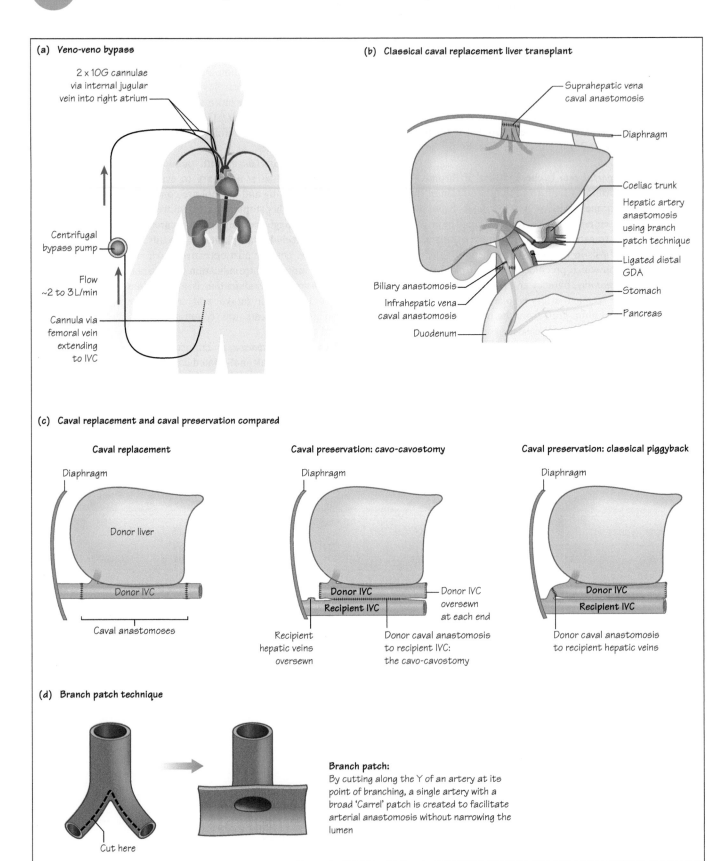

(a) Veno-veno bypass

2 x 10G cannulae via internal jugular vein into right atrium

Centrifugal bypass pump

Flow ~2 to 3 L/min

Cannula via femoral vein extending to IVC

(b) Classical caval replacement liver transplant

Suprahepatic vena caval anastomosis

Diaphragm

Coeliac trunk

Hepatic artery anastomosis using branch patch technique

Ligated distal GDA

Stomach

Pancreas

Biliary anastomosis

Infrahepatic vena caval anastomosis

Duodenum

(c) Caval replacement and caval preservation compared

Caval replacement

Diaphragm

Donor liver

Donor IVC

Caval anastomoses

Caval preservation: cavo-cavostomy

Diaphragm

Donor IVC

Recipient IVC

Donor IVC oversewn at each end

Recipient hepatic veins oversewn

Donor caval anastomosis to recipient IVC: the cavo-cavostomy

Caval preservation: classical piggyback

Diaphragm

Donor IVC

Recipient IVC

Donor caval anastomosis to recipient hepatic veins

(d) Branch patch technique

Cut here

Branch patch:
By cutting along the Y of an artery at its point of branching, a single artery with a broad 'Carrel' patch is created to facilitate arterial anastomosis without narrowing the lumen

Transplantation at a Glance, First Edition. Menna Clatworthy, Christopher Watson, Michael Allison and John Dark.

Liver transplantation is an extreme surgical undertaking, both for the patient and the surgical team. There are two components to the operation.

Recipient hepatectomy

Portal hypertension, vascular adhesions from previous surgery and coagulopathy make removing a cirrhotic liver a bloody affair.

As the abdomen is opened care must be taken not to damage a recannalised para-umbilical vein if present, which shunts blood from the liver to the umbilicus, where it feeds the caput medusa.

The principles of hepatectomy are to divide the bile duct, hepatic artery and portal vein close to the hilum, leaving good lengths of vessels for subsequent anastomosis. The bile duct is divided first, then the hepatic artery. The portal vein may be left in continuity until the liver is fully mobilised, or it may be divided and joined end-to-side to the vena cava forming a temporary porto-caval shunt which decompresses the portal hypertension, reducing blood loss.

The peritoneal attachments of the liver are divided, freeing the left lobe and mobilising the right lobe's 'bare area' from the diaphragm.

The liver sits astride the inferior vena cava (IVC), and can be removed either with or without the 'intrahepatic' portion of IVC. The IVC must be removed if there is a tumour in close proximity to it; otherwise it may be left in situ and the liver removed from the IVC. This is done by dividing the small and multiple veins from the caudate lobe which drain directly into the anterior surface of the IVC, and then dividing the right, middle and left hepatic vein. Leaving the IVC has the advantage of maintaining venous return to the heart and not compromising renal vein outflow. Where the IVC is removed it may be necessary to place the patient on a veno-veno bypass circuit that shunts blood from the IVC below (via a femoral vein cannula) to the superior vena cava (SVC) above (via an axillary or internal jugular vein cannula). Typically flows of 2 to 3 litres/min are achieved in such a circuit.

Implantation of the new liver

The new liver usually requires minor surgery to make it transplant-able. The phrenic veins that drain into the suprahepatic IVC are oversewn lest they bleed on reperfusion. The hepatic artery is isolated, as is the portal vein, to facilitate subsequent anastomosis; any branches are ligated.

Caval anastomoses

Caval replacement: where the IVC has been removed with the old liver, the new liver is implanted by sewing the upper and lower ends of the IVC to the corresponding parts of the donor liver.

Caval conservation: where the IVC has been left in continuity, the new liver can be anastomosed either by sewing the suprahe-patic IVC of the donor to the confluence of the recipient's three hepatic veins which are opened out into one ('classical piggyback'), or after oversewing the supra- and infrahepatic donor IVC, by sewing the anterior aspect of the recipient IVC to the posterior aspect of the donor IVC (cavo-cavostomy).

Portal vein anastomosis

The portal vein is usually joined directly to the new portal vein. If the recipient's portal vein is thrombosed, a length of donor iliac vein may be used to join the donor portal vein to the recipient's superior mesenteric vein.

Hepatic artery anastomosis

To avoid narrowing the artery at the anastomosis, it is usually performed at the site of branching where the diameter may be made larger; typical sites are the recipient hepatic artery or gas-troduodenal artery bifurcation to the donor coeliac trunk or splenic artery bifurcation (*see* Figure 34). If the recipient artery is blocked then a length of donor iliac artery is used to provide a conduit to either the supracoeliac or infrarenal aorta.

Bile duct anastomosis

Simple end-to-end anastomosis is most commonly performed. Where there is a large size discrepancy, or prior duct disease (such as in primary sclerosing cholangitis or cystic fibrosis), the donor bile duct is joined to a length of jejunum (hepatico-jejunostomy) fashioned into a Roux-en-Y loop.

Closure

Since the liver produces most of the coagulation factors, the patient will usually need third-party clotting factors in the form of fresh frozen plasma during the hepatectomy and while anhepatic. Following reperfusion with recipient blood the new liver takes some time to produce its own clotting factors, so bleeding is common. Therefore it is important to pay careful attention to stopping all bleeding points before closing the abdomen, since they are unlikely to stop bleeding by themselves. Where there is signifi-cant ongoing bleeding it may be necessary to pack the liver with swabs and return 48 hours later to remove them, by which time the clotting should have returned to normal.

Split liver or live donor transplantation

The liver may be divided in a live donor, removing either the right lobe for another adult or the left lobe for a child. In the case of a deceased donor the splitting takes place on a back table, with the liver immersed in ice-cold preservation solution, producing part of a liver for each of two recipients. The surgeon then has half a liver to implant.

The left lateral segment for a child typically has just the left hepatic vein and left branches of the artery, portal vein and bile duct. The recipient's vena cava is left in place and the liver placed on top of it.

A right lobe, which may or may not contain segment IV, has the donor vena cava and can be implanted with either caval conserva-tion or caval replacement techniques. Whenever the liver is split there is an increased chance of 'small for size', where the liver substance is insufficient for the recipient, a situation that may be made worse by the longer cold ischaemia experienced when having to first split the liver. Transplantation of the right lobe from a split liver is associated with a 1.5 times greater risk of graft failure compared with using the whole liver; the extra risk is offset by being able to treat a child and adult with the same liver.

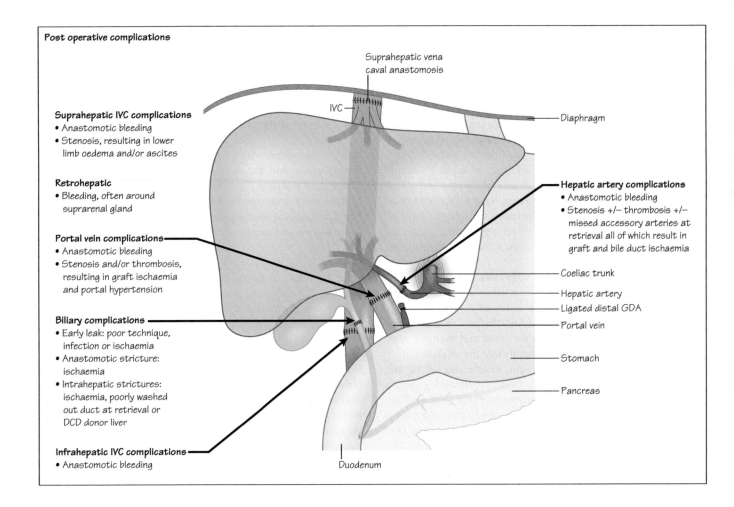

Post operative complications

Suprahepatic IVC complications
- Anastomotic bleeding
- Stenosis, resulting in lower limb oedema and/or ascites

Retrohepatic
- Bleeding, often around suprarenal gland

Portal vein complications
- Anastomotic bleeding
- Stenosis and/or thrombosis, resulting in graft ischaemia and portal hypertension

Biliary complications
- Early leak: poor technique, infection or ischaemia
- Anastomotic stricture: ischaemia
- Intrahepatic strictures: ischaemia, poorly washed out duct at retrieval or DCD donor liver

Infrahepatic IVC complications
- Anastomotic bleeding

Suprahepatic vena caval anastomosis

IVC

Diaphragm

Hepatic artery complications
- Anastomotic bleeding
- Stenosis +/− thrombosis +/− missed accessory arteries at retrieval all of which result in graft and bile duct ischaemia

Coeliac trunk

Hepatic artery

Ligated distal GDA

Portal vein

Stomach

Pancreas

Duodenum

Monitoring the liver

Careful and frequent clinical review is required post transplant to identify deterioration suggestive of complications. Post-transplant biochemical monitoring uses the same markers of liver dysfunction as were used before transplantation, namely:
- prothrombin time, for synthetic function;
- alanine transaminase (ALT) and aspartate transaminase (AST), for hepatocellular damage;
- alkaline phosphatase (ALP): reflects bile duct damage;
- serum lactate, should start to fall towards normal within an hour or two of reperfusion of the liver giving earliest sign of function;
- ultrasonography is used to detect biliary dilatation and assess blood flow to the liver, supplemented by CT angiography.

Surgical complications

Non-specific complications of surgery

Bleeding is common due to a combination of factors:
- the presence of abdominal varices
- a coagulopathy, particularly if the liver is slow to resume full protein synthesis
- thrombocytopaenia due to splenomegaly
- multiple venous and arterial anastomoses.

Wound infection is common due to the prolonged nature of the surgery (many hours), the poor nutritional state of the recipient and the reaccumulation of ascites post-operatively.

Wound breakdown, with superficial or complete dehiscence, may follow.

Atelectasis, pneumonia and pleural effusion are also common, as with all upper abdominal surgery, and occasionally paralysis of the right hemidiaphragm occurs as a consequence of cross-clamping the suprahepatic vena cava alongside which runs the right phrenic nerve.

Biliary complications

The bile duct is the commonest source of problems following transplantation. In part this relates to its blood supply, which usually passes from the duodenal end of the duct towards the liver; the common hepatic duct and confluence receive a blood supply from the common or right hepatic artery. Following transplant the only blood supply to the bile duct is from the liver and so it is prone to ischaemia unless cut short; if cut too short the ensuing anastomosis is under tension, which predisposes to anastomotic disruption.

Bile leak may occur as a result of ischaemia, infection or traction on the anastomosis. It commonly affects a duct-to-duct anasto-

Transplantation at a Glance, First Edition. Menna Clatworthy, Christopher Watson, Michael Allison and John Dark.

78 © 2012 John Wiley & Sons, Ltd. Published 2012 by John Wiley & Sons, Ltd.

mosis and requires conversion to a Roux-en-Y choledocho-jejunostomy. Since it may signify stenosis or thrombosis of the main or accessory right hepatic artery this should be excluded before surgery.

Anastomotic stricture may occur, usually as a result of ischaemia. Diagnosis is suggested by raised bilirubin and ALP, with dilated bile ducts on ultrasound. The stricture may be confirmed on magnetic resonance imaging followed by endoscopic retrograde cholangio-pancreatography (ERCP), balloon angioplasty and stenting. Persistent strictures may require conversion to Roux-en-Y drainage.

Arterial complications

Hepatic artery thrombosis early post-transplant usually manifests with a sudden clinical deterioration and concomitant worsening of liver biochemistry. Thrombosis in the late post-operative period, months or years after transplant, may present more insidiously with biliary complications (intrahepatic strictures) or liver abscess formation.

Hepatic artery stenosis may also present with biliary complications in the early post-transplant period.

Venous outflow

Venous outflow problems are usually secondary to a suprahepatic vena caval anastomotic stenosis where a classical caval replacement technique has been used for transplant. Presentation is with marked ascites and lower limb oedema. Diagnosis is by measurement of a pressure gradient across the anastomosis, and balloon angioplasty is the treatment of choice.

Portal venous inflow

Portal vein thrombosis is unusual but may occur early post-transplant, particular in patients with a prior portal or mesenteric venous thrombosis.

Medical complications

As with post-operative surgical complications, the medical complications of liver transplantation can be early or late. All the well-recognised general medical complications seen after major surgery, including myocardial infarction/cardiac decompensation, chest sepsis, confusion, electrolyte disturbances and renal dysfunction, can also occur post-liver transplantation.

In addition, in keeping with other transplants, acute rejection is common in the early post-transplant period but rarely causes long-term damage. Rejection is usually cell-mediated, although antibody-mediated rejection may also occur.

Recurrent disease

Hepatocellular tumours may recur following transplant, as well as other liver diseases, including:

Hepatitis C

Hepatitis C virus (HCV) invariably infects the transplanted liver and can result in aggressive disease, such that up to 10% of patients develop graft failure within a year post-transplant and around 30% develop cirrhosis in the transplanted liver within 5 years. Antiviral treatment can be used to modify the prognosis of hepatitis C post-transplant.

Hepatitis B

Hepatitis B can infect the transplanted liver, although the combination of regular infusions of hepatitis B immune globulin (HBIG) together with HBV replication inhibitors, such as lamivudine, usually controls disease.

Autoimmune disease

Primary biliary cirrhosis, autoimmune hepatitis and primary sclerosing cholangitis are all recognised to recur in a minority of liver transplant recipients.

Alcoholic liver disease

Alcohol-related liver disease (ALD) and non-alcoholic fatty liver disease can also recur post transplant, although steps are taken pre-transplant to attempt to determine those ALD patients who are at high risk of harmful drinking post transplant and thereby reduce disease recurrence.

Long-term outcomes

With good short-term outcomes following liver transplantation, the aim is to reduce long-term morbidity. To that end, every effort is made to minimise cardiovascular risk factors (treating hypertension, hyperlipidaemia and diabetes), to recognise disease recurrence early and to limit renal toxicity by using low doses of calcineurin inhibitor or converting to non-nephrotoxic agents such as mTOR inhibitors.

Long-term survival after liver transplantation is good, with more than 90% of recipients surviving a year and 70% more than 5 years.

(a) Diseases requiring intestinal transplantation according to international registry

Disease	Children (%)	Adult (%)
Short bowel syndrome		
Volvulus	17	7
Gastroschisis	21	1
Trauma	2	8
Necrotising enterocolitis	13	1
Ischaemia	1	25
Crohn's disease	–	12
Intestinal atresia	8	–
Other	2	8
Malabsorption		
Microvillous inclusion	6	–
Other	2	–
Motility disorder		
Pseudo-obstruction	9	9
Aganglionosis	8	–
Other	1	–
Tumours (e.g. desmoid)	1	15
Retransplantation	8	7
Other	2	5

(b) Indications for transplantation

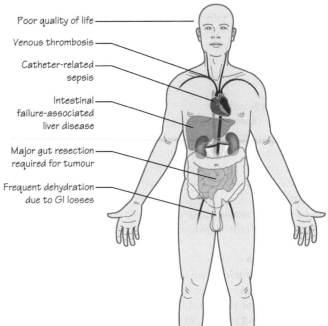

Poor quality of life

Venous thrombosis

Catheter-related sepsis

Intestinal failure-associated liver disease

Major gut resection required for tumour

Frequent dehydration due to GI losses

(c) Assessment for transplantation

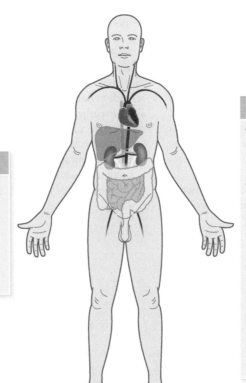

Specific questions to address

- **Duplex/MR venography**
  - What veins are present?
- **Liver:** ultrasound; biochemistry, biopsy:
  - Is there evidence of IFALD?
- **Abdominal domain**
  - How much space is there in the abdomen?

Standard screening tests

- **Cardiac**
  - ECG
  - Echo
  - Stress MPI/echo
- **Respiratory**
  - Lung capacity
  - Gas transfer
- **Endoscopy**
  - oesophagus, stomach and duodenum plus biopsies
- **CT/barium studies**
  - Length of existing bowel
- **If tumour**
  - Staging CT abdomen and chest
- **Renal function**
  - Biochemistry and GFR measurement
- **Virology screen**

Transplantation at a Glance, First Edition. Menna Clatworthy, Christopher Watson, Michael Allison and John Dark.

80 © 2012 John Wiley & Sons, Ltd. Published 2012 by John Wiley & Sons, Ltd.

Intestinal failure

Intestinal failure means that the patient can no longer maintain their nutritional needs by oral intake of food. In some patients, for example those who have had a recent bowel resection, this is a temporary state that will recover as the residual bowel adapts; in others with very diseased bowel or major resections the condition may be irreversible with a continued requirement for parenteral nutrition (PN).

Parenteral nutrition is the main treatment for patients with intestinal failure. It requires an indwelling central venous catheter to which the patient connects a bag of nutrition (typically 2.5 litres) every evening to run over 12 to 14 hours through the night. Most patients can live a reasonable existence on such therapy.

Complications of parenteral nutrition

The 1-year survival of a patient on home PN is 90%, falling to 65% at 5 years. There are three principal complications of long-term PN.

Catheter-related sepsis

The central venous catheter may become infected during the course of setting up or taking down the PN infusion, or if the catheter is damaged. Sepsis may remain line-associated or may result in infective endocarditis or other disseminated infection.

Venous thrombosis

Indwelling cannulas are associated with venous thrombosis, with loss of that central vein for future access. Patients predisposed to thrombosis may rapidly lose their internal jugular veins or even thrombose the superior vena cava (SVC), necessitating a cannula in a femoral vein or, via direct translumbar puncture, in the inferior vena cava (IVC). Extensive venous thrombosis may preclude transplantation, so early referral as venous access diminishes is important.

Intestinal failure associated liver disease (IFALD)

Liver disease affects over half of patients on long-term PN, although it may start before PN is instituted in the very malnourished patient. In children, this is commonly due to cholestasis, in adults it is usually steatohepatitis. Steatohepatitis is probably a consequence of the high glucose intake, stimulating insulin production which promotes lipogenesis, combined with high lipid infusions. In both groups the disease may progress to fibrosis and cirrhosis.

Biliary sludge and gallstones are common in both age groups, and is associated with short bowel syndrome in the absence of PN.

Other factors predicting poor outcome on PN

The other factors associated with a poor outcome on PN are age (children, and adults over 60); extremely short length of residual bowel (<50 cm); dysmotility disorders; radiation enteritis; and longer duration of treatment.

Indications for transplantation

Intestinal transplantation is indicated for one of three main reasons.
1 Complications of parenteral nutrition (PN):
  • PN-induced liver injury;
  • thrombosis of two or more central veins;
  • two or more episodes of catheter-related sepsis per year requiring hospitalisation;
  • a single episode of fungal catheter-related sepsis; septic shock;
  • frequent severe dehydration due to gut losses despite intravenous fluid supplementation and PN.

2 Requirement for major gut resection for tumour, such as a desmoid tumour invading the mesentery.
3 Unacceptable quality of life on PN.

Assessment for transplantation

There are three main aspects to the assessment of intestinal transplant recipients.

Fitness for surgery

Multivisceral transplantation is akin to liver transplantation in its surgical stress. Full cardiological and respiratory assessments are performed. Since kidney failure is common post-intestinal transplantation and is difficult to assess in patients on PN, a nuclear medicine glomerular filtration rate (GFR) measurement is required to gauge the need for simultaneous kidney transplantation.

Extensive venous mapping is usually required to identify sites for peri-operative access. The presence of SVC thrombosis is a contraindication to a liver transplant using a classical caval replacement technique, because this would remove all venous return to the heart. At least one femoral vein needs to be patent, with patency of the IVC.

A preferred site for a stoma should be marked, and the patient should receive appropriate stoma counselling.

Patients undergoing modified or full multivisceral transplantation will undergo splenectomy as part of the explant procedure. They should therefore be immunised against meningococcus, pneumococcus and haemophilus influenza before listing.

Extensive psychological assessment is required, particularly of anyone undergoing the procedure only for quality-of-life.

Liver disease

Is there any evidence of underlying liver disease? Imaging, including duplex ultrasound of the liver, and liver biopsy are usually required in addition to liver biochemistry to assess whether the liver is affected by IFALD, and if so, whether it needs replacing.

Surgical anatomy

Previous surgical history detailing any and every resection is important to enable judgement as to what is feasible. This is supplemented by contrast imaging of the remaining bowel, together with endoscopic inspection of any bowel to be left in situ to exclude disease, and also inspection of any bowel to be removed to confirm the diagnosis if required.

Three-dimensional imaging of the gut is particularly important in the case of malignancy to allow estimation of the extent of the tumour. Desmoids, the commonest malignancy for which transplantation is undertaken, are associated with intestinal polyposis (Gardner syndrome) and usually arise within the mesentery and extend to the adjacent structures, such as the abdominal wall, renal tract or great vessels in the retroperitoneum. All residual tumour should be removed.

Results of intestinal transplantation

Outcomes following intestinal transplantation vary, and are better in centres with high-volume programmes, in younger recipients and in patients transplanted from home rather than in those who were inpatients already. Overall graft survival rates are around 80% and patient survival rates are around 90% at 1 year.

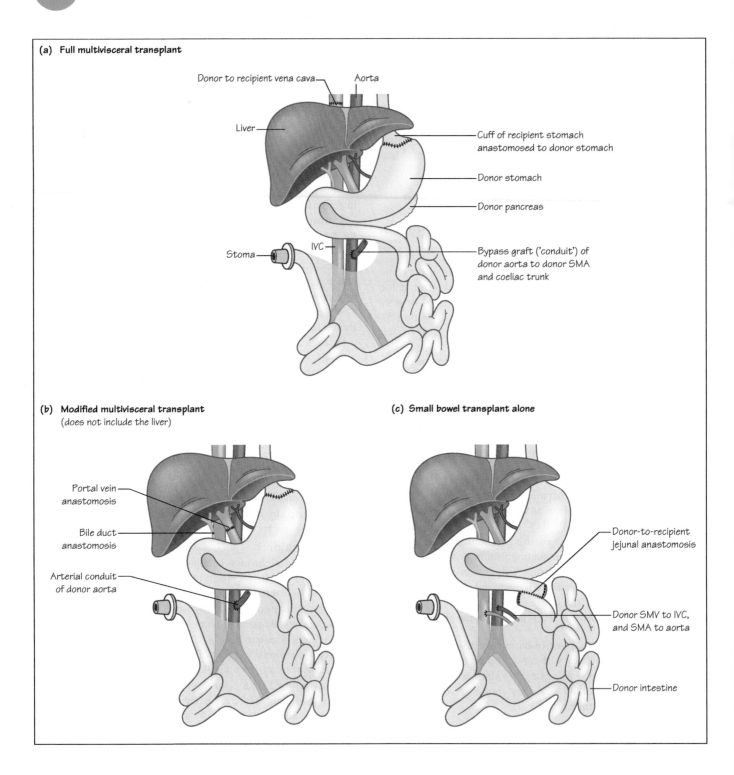

(a) Full multivisceral transplant

Donor to recipient vena cava

Aorta

Liver

Cuff of recipient stomach anastomosed to donor stomach

Donor stomach

Donor pancreas

Stoma

IVC

Bypass graft ('conduit') of donor aorta to donor SMA and coeliac trunk

(b) Modified multivisceral transplant
(does not include the liver)

Portal vein anastomosis

Bile duct anastomosis

Arterial conduit of donor aorta

(c) Small bowel transplant alone

Donor-to-recipient jejunal anastomosis

Donor SMV to IVC, and SMA to aorta

Donor intestine

Types of transplant

There are three main types of intestinal transplantation performed. All involve transplanting a sufficient length of small intestine to achieve independence from parenteral nutrition (PN). The large intestine is not usually transplanted, although its inclusion has been proposed as a way to reduce fluid losses. The terminal ileum is brought out as an ileostomy to facilitate biopsy, although this may be reversed in the long term by anastomosis to the native

Transplantation at a Glance, First Edition. Menna Clatworthy, Christopher Watson, Michael Allison and John Dark.

colon (if still present) to restore gut continuity. Where there is pre-existing renal failure it is sensible to perform a kidney transplant at the same time.

Other operative combinations are possible (such as liver and small bowel alone), but the three below are the most common.

Multivisceral transplant

Where there is intestinal failure and severe associated liver disease, it is customary to perform a transplant that includes liver and small bowel; this is most easily accomplished by implanting a bloc of tissue (a cluster) which also includes the stomach, duodenum and pancreas, and which receives its arterial supply from the coeliac trunk and superior mesenteric artery (SMA), with venous drainage via the hepatic veins with the liver implanted either using the caval replacement or piggyback technique (see Chapter 35). The donor stomach is anastomosed to a cuff of recipient stomach just below the diaphragmatic hiatus.

The transplanted stomach is denervated, so the vagus nerve supply is absent, resulting in closure of the pylorus, which prevents gastric emptying. A gastric drainage procedure is therefore necessary, either a pyloroplasty or a gastroenterostomy.

Modified multivisceral transplant

Where the liver is minimally diseased with an anticipation of recovery, a transplant excluding liver is appropriate. If there has been previous gastric or pancreatic disease, such as PN-related pancreatitis, the bloc of tissue should include the stomach and duodenum, with the portal vein being anastomosed to the recipient portal vein at the hilum of the liver.

Small bowel alone

Isolated small bowel transplantation is the simplest procedure to undergo. The SMA is anastomosed to the aorta, the superior mesenteric vein (SMV) to the inferior vena cava (IVC); if the liver function is satisfactory there is no need for a portal venous anastomosis.

An isolated intestinal transplant has the additional advantage that, should serious complications occur, it can be readily removed and the patient returned to PN until fit for a retransplant.

Donor assessment

Since the majority of patients undergoing intestinal transplantation have had multiple bowel resections there is very little peritoneal cavity remaining (known as abdominal domain). Donor organs therefore need to be smaller than the recipient wherever possible, to enable closure of the abdomen.

Aside from the issues of size, the donor organs are generally best obtained from slim individuals with little mesenteric fat in order to facilitate rapid cooling on retrieval.

Operative issues
Anaesthetic concerns
1 *Volume replacement*: requires at least one large-volume line.
2 *For veno-veno bypass* where caval replacement or cross-clamping of the IVC is involved, a patient central vein above the diaphragm is necessary.
3 *Reperfusion of multivisceral block* can release a large volume of cold potassium-rich preservation solution, which precipitates cardiac arrest.

Surgical issues
1 *Abdominal domain*: is there sufficient space in the abdomen to fit the new intestine/bloc of tissue? It is undesirable to leave the abdomen open, although sometimes necessary in small children.
2 *Arterial inflow to the graft* is via an SMA anastomosis on to the infrarenal aorta in an isolated graft; for a multivisceral graft a conduit of donor aorta is used to take blood from the infrarenal aorta to the SMA and coeliac trunk. It is undesirable to clamp the aorta above the renal arteries because of the renal ischaemia this causes.
3 *A gastric drainage procedure*, such as a pyloroplasty, is required when the stomach is part of the multivisceral bloc.
4 *Tolerance of the intestine to cold ischaemia* is much more critical than that of the liver or kidney. It is desirable to reperfuse the intestinal bloc within 4 hours where possible, although inevitably this is a compromise between proximity of the donor and difficulties encountered during the operation to prepare the recipient to take the bloc, an operation that may take many hours.

Post-transplant complications
Peri-operative complications
1 *Thrombosis of arterial supply or venous drainage* is a risk, because many of the recipients have lost their original bowel due to a procoagulant tendency. In some cases this will have been cured by replacement of the liver.
2 *Delayed resumption of normal bowel function* is common. The stomach is the last organ to start to work, often taking more than 3 weeks before peristalsis starts and it empties. Nutrition during this time is achieved using a jejunostomy into the new bowel.

Transplantation related complications
1 *Rejection* is more common than with other organs, hence enhanced immunosuppression is required. Typical presentations are with increased or decreased bowel activity, with sepsis a common feature. The latter is a consequence of rejection impairing the mucosal barrier and permitting translocation of bacteria. The result is a need to enhance immunosuppression in a septic patient.
2 *Infection* is common, and often associated with intestinal rejection or intra-abdominal collections.
3 *Renal impairment*. Intestinal transplant recipients have the highest incidence of kidney failure of any non-renal transplant type. This is in part due to the high-volume fluid losses from the gut, as well as the nephrotoxic immunosuppression.
4 *Recurrent disease*, such as Crohn's disease, may occur.
5 *Graft versus host disease* is more likely after a multivisceral transplant than other forms of solid organ transplant and tends to occur within the first 3 or 4 months. This is because of the large amount of lymphoid tissue (mesenteric lymph nodes and mucosa-associated lymphoid tissue) in the graft, particularly if the donor spleen has been transplanted, as used to occur in some centres in the US. Lymphocytes transplanted with the donor can 'reject' the recipient, rather than the other way around. Features include perfect function of the donor organs, but rash, impaired liver function (only if liver is not part of graft) and fever. It is fatal in a significant proportion of those affected.

(a) Indications for heart transplantation in the UK (2008–10)

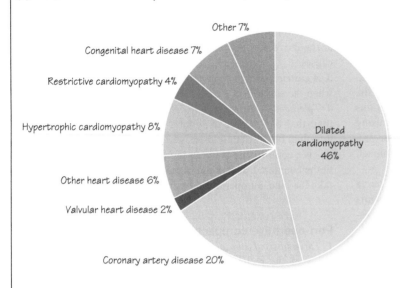

- Other 7%
- Congenital heart disease 7%
- Restrictive cardiomyopathy 4%
- Hypertrophic cardiomyopathy 8%
- Other heart disease 6%
- Valvular heart disease 2%
- Coronary artery disease 20%
- Dilated cardiomyopathy 46%

(b) The Frank–Starling relationship

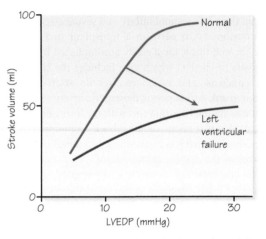

Normal

Stroke volume (ml)

Left ventricular failure

LVEDP (mmHg)

Loss of contractility in heart failure leads to a down-shift in the Frank–Starling curve. Much higher LVEDP are required to increase stroke volume (and hence cardiac output)

(c) Assessment for heart transplantation

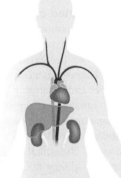

Comorbidity

- Smoking
- Recent pulmonary embolism
- Lung disease
  - FEV_1 or FVC <50% predicted
- Obesity (BMI: 30 kg/m^2)
- Hepatitis C, HIV
- Renal dysfunction
- Diabetes mellitus with complications
- Recent history of cancer (within 5 years)
- Peripheral vascular disease

Investigations

- Right heart catheter:
  - PA pressure
  - Pulmonary vascular resistance
  - Transpulmonary gradient
- Cardiopulmonary exercise test: determine peak VO$_2$
- History: NYHA grade

(d) Cardiopulmonary exercise testing

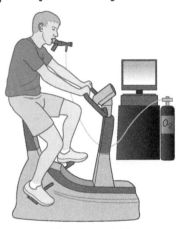

Inspired and expired O_2 and expired CO_2 are measured during progressively increasing exercise to evaluate peak O_2 consumption (VO$_2$ max)

(e) New York Heart Association Functional Classification

NYHA class	Symptoms
I	No symptoms, no limitation in ordinary physical activity (e.g. shortness of breath on walking, climbing stairs)
II	Mild symptoms (SOB, angina) and slight limitation of ordinary activity
III	Marked limitation in activity due to symptoms, with minimal activity (e.g. walking 20–100 m). Comfortable only at rest
IV	Severe limitation. Symptoms even while at rest. Often bedbound

While heart transplantation remains an excellent treatment for advanced heart failure, the number of transplants performed in Europe is falling due to the lack of suitable donors. The assessment of potential recipients has therefore become more stringent in order to make optimal use of available organs. Many patients referred for transplantation can be improved with conventional cardiac surgery and/or improved medical management, including resynchronisation therapy with biventricular pacing. A classification of underlying diseases is given in Figure 39.

Assessment for transplantation
The assessment of potential recipients involves three components:
- functional capacity
- right heart catheterisation to assess pulmonary circulation
- comorbidity.

Evaluating functional capacity
Functional capacity can be partly assessed by the history (NYHA classification grade IV), but accurate quantification usually relies on cardiopulmonary exercise testing (CPET).

CPET involves accurate measurements of inspired and expired O_2, expired CO_2, minute ventilation and work done, typically while using a bicycle ergometer. The maximal oxygen uptake (VO_2 peak) is usually that measured at the termination of exercise.

The CPET allows patients to be divided into three prognostic categories, providing full medical therapy, including beta-blockade, has been prescribed.
1 Peak VO_2 <12 ml/kg/min with no contraindications to heart transplantation: 94% 1-year survival.
2 Peak VO_2 <12 ml/kg/min with some contraindications to heart transplantation: 74% 1-year survival.
3 Peak VO_2 >12 ml/kg/min: 47% 1-year survival.

Evaluating the pulmonary circulation
Chronic left ventricular failure is characterised by a loss of myocardial contractility and higher left ventricular diastolic pressures (LVEDP) in an effort to maintain cardiac output. Raised LVEDP leads to an increase in pulmonary venous pressure and pulmonary artery (PA) pressure. The rise in PA pressure is accompanied by a rise in pulmonary vascular resistance (PVR).

Raised PVR is usually reversible following transplantation, but can cause acute right ventricular failure in the newly transplanted heart, and accounts for 20% of early deaths post-transplant. Therefore a high pulmonary artery pressure (>60 mmHg), high transpulmonary pressure gradient (TPG >15 mmHg), and high PVR (>5 Wood units) are contraindications to heart transplantation. To assess these values patients undergo right heart catheterisation using a Swan–Ganz catheter. The PVR can be improved by increasing diuretics and other anti-failure treatments. It should be regularly re-assessed while awaiting transplant.

Evaluating comorbidity
Patients with previous cardiac surgery (congenital heart disease, previous coronary artery bypass graft [CABG] or valve surgery, previous heart transplant) have a higher morbidity and mortality related to adhesions and disruption of tissue planes.

Age – older patients have a poorer outcome, although chronological age per se is not a contraindication if the patient is otherwise fit. Transplantation is rarely offered to patients ≥70 years.

Smoking – smokers have a reduced survival, with a higher incidence of cardiac allograft vasculopathy.

Cerebrovascular or peripheral vascular disease if symptomatic.

Lung disease – severe lung disease, with FEV_1 and FVC <50% predicted.

Thromboembolic disease – recent pulmonary embolism is a contraindication (raises PA pressure and may proceed to lung abscess post-operatively).

Diabetes mellitus with severe end organ damage, e.g. nephropathy.

Kidney function – renal function is often affected by heart failure, and will be affected by the immunosuppression following surgery. In general, a glomerular filtration rate (GFR) above 40 ml/min/1.73m^2 is considered adequate. Patients with poor renal function might be considered for later kidney transplant. Combined heart and kidney transplantation is now not normally done because of the excessive morbidity of two procedures.

Infection – active infection, or chronic viral infections (e.g. HIV, hepatitis C virus).

Malignancy – a recent history of cancer (except non-melanoma skin cancer) is a contraindication. A recurrence-free interval of 5 years is appropriate before transplantation might be considered.

Obesity – obese patients have increased morbidity and mortality, so patients with a BMI >30 kg/m^2 are usually excluded.

Poor compliance – substance abuse, inability to stop smoking or a history of poor adherence to drug treatment are all predictors of a bad outcome due to inability to follow immunosuppressive drug regimens.

Bridge to transplantation
Many patients who have been deemed suitable for heart transplantation have such poor hearts that they are unlikely to survive the wait for a suitable heart, in spite of inotrope support on an intensive care unit. To support such hearts during this time increasing use is being made of mechanical circulatory support in the form of ventricular assist devices (VADs). These devices provide an additional pump to aid the circulation. The standard configuration is a pump draining blood from the apex of the left ventricle and returning it via a tube graft to the ascending aorta. This left-sided – LVAD –support is generally sufficient; the requirement for support of both ventricles predicts a much worse outcome.

In the short term, the very sick patient can be stabilised with externally placed (paracorporeal) pumps which give pulsatile flow. Longer-term support is best given by fully implanted miniature centrifugal, continuous-flow pumps. The current generation lies entirely within the pericardial cavity. Although there remain some unsolved problems of biocompatibility, particularly thrombosis, the need for rigorous anticoagulant control and infection, the 1-year survival, at 80–85%, is similar to heart transplantation. The future treatment for the very large number of patients with end-stage heart failure will be with these mechanical devices and their successors.

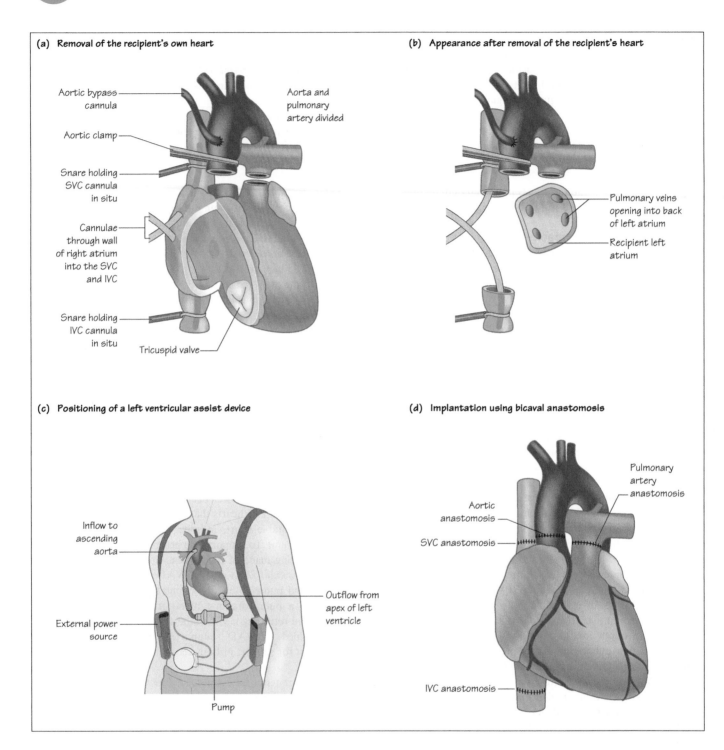

(a) **Removal of the recipient's own heart**

Aortic bypass cannula

Aortic clamp

Snare holding SVC cannula in situ

Cannulae through wall of right atrium into the SVC and IVC

Snare holding IVC cannula in situ

Tricuspid valve

Aorta and pulmonary artery divided

(b) **Appearance after removal of the recipient's heart**

Pulmonary veins opening into back of left atrium

Recipient left atrium

(c) **Positioning of a left ventricular assist device**

Inflow to ascending aorta

External power source

Outflow from apex of left ventricle

Pump

(d) **Implantation using bicaval anastomosis**

Pulmonary artery anastomosis

Aortic anastomosis

SVC anastomosis

IVC anastomosis

Transplantation at a Glance, First Edition. Menna Clatworthy, Christopher Watson, Michael Allison and John Dark.

Donor selection
Waiting list mortality
The appropriateness of using any organ for transplantation must be balanced against the risk of the recipient dying on the waiting list if the transplant does not proceed, and in the knowledge that many other patients who might potentially benefit from transplantation have been excluded from the list because of donor organ shortage. In the first year on the waiting list around 60% of patients will receive a heart, while 10–15% will die waiting.

Suitable hearts
As with all organs, donor sepsis and current or recent malignancy are contraindications, apart from primary intracranial malignancy. The heart must be ABO-compatible and lacking HLA antigens to which the recipient has pre-existent antibodies; 30–40% of recipients are sensitised in this fashion.

Other considerations include the following.
- *Donor age:* older donors have an increased burden of coronary artery disease, and donors over 55 years are seldom used.
- *Donor coronary artery disease* is associated with early graft failure, unless corrective surgery is performed to bypass the donor coronary arteries.
- *Donor valvular disease or significant left ventricular hypertrophy.* Echocardiography is a useful way to identify diseased valves (some of which can be repaired) and left ventricular hypertrophy. A septal thickness of >1.6 cm is a contraindication to donation.
- *Death from carbon monoxide* poisoning with carboxyhaemoglobin level above 20%.
- *Donor size:* aim is to use hearts from donors with similar weight to recipient; smaller donor hearts and hearts from females, particularly for recipients with pulmonary hypertension, tend to fare poorly.
- *Left ventricular dysfunction* is a common complication of brainstem death, probably related to the catecholamine storm that occurs. With time and donor fluid management some of these hearts will recover and be suitable for transplantation; severe dysfunction (hypokinesia, arrhythmia) is a contraindication.

The donor heart must be macroscopically examined by the retrieving surgeon. In addition, measurement of cardiac output and left-side filling pressures, usually with a Swan–Ganz catheter is an essential part of donor assessment.

Transplanting the heart
Removing the recipient heart
The heart is approached through a midline incision dividing the sternum along its length, a median sternotomy. The recipient is placed on cardiopulmonary bypass so the oxygenation and pump functions are provided. Cannulae are placed in the ascending aorta and separate cannulae in the superior and inferior vena cavae.

Blood is then pumped from the vena cavae to the bypass machine and back into the aortic cannula, and the patient is cooled to 30°C.

When the donor heart is within 20 minutes of the recipient centre the recipient's heart is removed. The aorta is cross-clamped and the cavae snared around the cannulae. The aorta and pulmonary arteries are divided just above the valves. Both cavae are divided to leave an adequate cuff for sewing to the donor right atrium. The left atrium is divided along the atrioventricular (AV) groove, leaving a cuff that contains all the pulmonary veins

Bi-caval implantation technique
The bi-caval implantation technique involves leaving the donor right atrium intact and instead performing separate anastomoses with the inferior vena cava (IVC) and superior vena cava (SVC). The benefits of having a normal size atrium include less atrial dysthyhmia, pacemaker requirement, tricuspid regurgitation and right ventricular dysfunction.

Additional considerations
Primary dysfunction of the donor heart is the cause of most early morbidity and mortality. Ischaemic time is very important. Mortality increases in a measurable fashion for every hour after the circulation stops. Good communication is essential between donor and recipient teams to minimise delays.

Previous cardiac surgery
Patients who have previously undergone a median sternotomy for cardiac surgery require much longer for cardiectomy, so it may be necessary to delay the explantation of the donor heart until the recipient team is ready.

Ventricular assist devices
These are removed at the start of the recipient procedure, after opening the chest, and may take additional time – 2 or 3 hours compared with the 20 minutes it takes to remove a 'normal' heart.

Congenital heart disease
The success of neonatal surgery for congenital heart disease has led to an increasing number of patients coming to require heart transplantation in later life. Many have unconventional anatomy, clear delineation of which is essential before surgery. Some procedures, such as in patients who have had surgery for transposition of the great vessels, may need cannulation of the femoral vessels instead to facilitate cardiopulmonary bypass. Additional lengths of aorta and SVC may be needed to cope with anatomical abnormalities. However, there is no condition, including dextrocardia, that precludes transplantation.

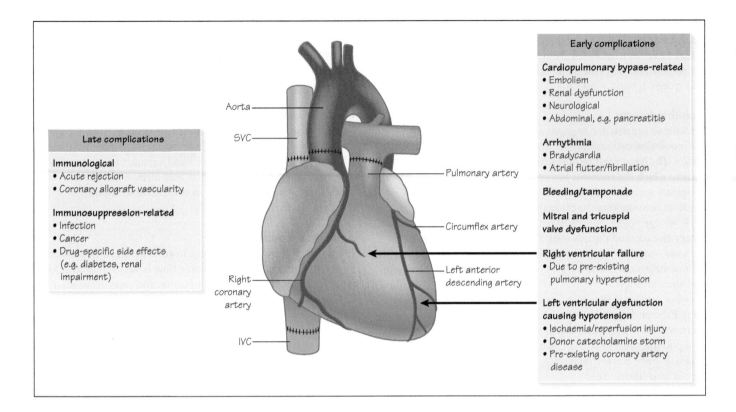

Late complications

Immunological
• Acute rejection
• Coronary allograft vascularity

Immunosuppression-related
• Infection
• Cancer
• Drug-specific side effects
  (e.g. diabetes, renal
  impairment)

Early complications

Cardiopulmonary bypass-related
• Embolism
• Renal dysfunction
• Neurological
• Abdominal, e.g. pancreatitis

Arrhythmia
• Bradycardia
• Atrial flutter/fibrillation

Bleeding/tamponade

**Mitral and tricuspid
valve dysfunction**

Right ventricular failure
• Due to pre-existing
  pulmonary hypertension

**Left ventricular dysfunction
causing hypotension**
• Ischaemia/reperfusion injury
• Donor catecholamine storm
• Pre-existing coronary artery
  disease

Labels: Aorta, SVC, Pulmonary artery, Circumflex artery, Left anterior descending artery, Right coronary artery, IVC

Early complications

The initial complications of heart transplantation relate to donor events, damage due to cold ischaemia, reperfusion injury, technical complications and the haemodynamic challenge facing the new heart in the recipient.

• *Bradycardia* – related to cold ischaemia, damage to the sino-atrial node or pre-transplant treatment with amiodarone. Treatment comprises either isoproterenol (isoprenaline) or temporary atrioventricular pacing.

• *Atrial fibrillation or flutter* occurs in up to a fifth of patients.

• *Right ventricular failure* – due to pre-existing pulmonary hypertension and high pulmonary vascular resistance. Isoproterenol is a pulmonary vasodilator as well as a chronotrope, and is used routinely. Inhaled nitric oxide can be a useful addition to reduce pulmonary artery pressure.

• *Systemic hypotension* may be due to impaired left ventricular function, which may recover. Reduction in peripheral vascular resistance may occur due to acidosis and vasoconstricting inotropes such as noradrenaline or vasopressin may be required.

• *Valvular dysfunction.* Tricuspid regurgitation is more common and may relate to dilatation of the tricuspid valve ring due to high pulmonary pressures. It typically recovers within 12 months.

• *Bleeding* resulting in tamponade may occur.

• *Pericardial effusion* may also occur and sometimes requires treatment, although it usually resolves within 6 weeks.

• *Renal* dysfunction is very common, particularly in patients with pre-existing renal impairment, those requiring prolonged bypass (retransplants, previous congenital heart disease) and as a consequence of calcineurin inhibitor immunosuppression. Short-term haemofiltration should be started early and does not confer any late disadvantage.

Immunosuppression

A typical immunosuppressive regimen would comprise an induction agent such as antithymocyte globulin or basiliximab, with maintenance therapy with tacrolimus, mycophenolate and steroids. In addition, statins such as pravastatin are also used in the early post-transplant period, regardless of serum cholesterol level.

Rejection

Hyperacute rejection

Hyperacute rejection is very uncommon. The short ischaemic tolerance of the heart means that formal cross-matching cannot usually be performed, and virtual cross-matching must be relied on. Transplantation in the presence of donor-specific antibody predicts less good outcome, with antibody-mediated rejection (AMR).

Acute rejection

Signs and symptoms of rejection are few, and the first presentation maybe with an arrhythmia. For this reason evidence of rejection is sought using frequent endocardial biospies. These are performed by passing fine biopsy forceps down the internal jugular vein and into the heart.

Most rejection is acute cellular rejection, which responds to pulsed high-dose steroids; AMR is increasingly being recognised.

Transplantation at a Glance, First Edition. Menna Clatworthy, Christopher Watson, Michael Allison and John Dark.

Cardiac allograft vasculopathy

Cardiac allograft vasculopathy (CAV) is the main cause of graft loss after the first year, with an incidence of around 50% at 10 years. It manifests as a diffuse accelerated form of atherosclerosis affecting the entire coronary arterial tree circumferentially, rather than appearing as the eccentric plaques in the large arteries that is typical of normal coronary artery disease.

Since the transplanted heart is denervated the recipient tends not to feel pain due to progressive ischaemia. Instead CAV is detected either on routine coronary angiography or the patient presents with new onset heart failure, arrhythmias, syncope or death. More recently intravascular ultrasound is being used to monitor the coronary arteries.

Treatment of CAV is preventative. Factors that might contribute to vascular disease, such as smoking, hypertension, diabetes and hyperlipidaemia are treated aggressively. In addition there is some evidence that the mTOR inhibitor immunosuppressants sirolimus and everolimus may prevent its occurrence.

Outcomes of heart transplantation

Current 1-year patient survival after a first heart transplant is 83%, with 60% surviving 10 years. The shortage of donor hearts, and the increased morbidity and mortality following retransplantation, means that most patients will not be considered for a second heart once the first heart fails.

(a) Indications for lung transplantation in the UK (2008–2010)

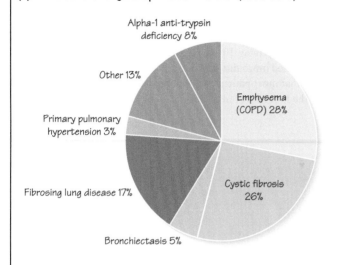

- Alpha-1 anti-trypsin deficiency 8%
- Other 13%
- Primary pulmonary hypertension 3%
- Fibrosing lung disease 17%
- Bronchiectasis 5%
- Cystic fibrosis 26%
- Emphysema (COPD) 28%

(b) The BODE index

Variable	Points			
	0	1	2	3
FEV$_1$ (% predicted)	≥65	50–64	36–49	≤35
6 – minute walk (metres)	≥350	250–349	150–249	≤149
Dyspnoea*	0–1	2	3	4
Body mass index	>21	≤21		

* Modified MRC dyspnoea scale

0 Breathless on strenous exercise

1 Breathless when hurrying on the level or walking up a slight incline

2 Walks slower than most people of the same age on the level because of breathlessness, or stops for breath while walking at own pace

3 Stop for breath after 100 metres or after a few minutes on the level

4 Too breathless to leave house or breathless when dressing

(c) Assessment for lung transplantation

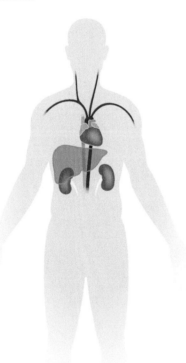

Comorbidity
• Smoking
• Hepatitis B, C, HIV
• Renal failure
• Diabetes mellitus with complications
• Recent history cancer (within 5 years)
• Peripheral vascular disease

Investigations

- 24–hour oesophageal pH ⎫ Exclude gastro-oesophageal
- Barium swallow ⎭ reflux disease

- FEV$_1$ – poor in COPD and CF
- FVC – poor in pulmonary fibrosis

- DLCO – poor in pulmonary fibrosis and COPD

- Body mass index ⎧ <18: malnourished – poor outcome
                    ⎩ >30: technically challenging surgery

- Bone density – poor in chronic lung disease and with long-term steroid usage

- PO$_2$; PCO$_2$ – hypoxaemia and hypercapnia

- 6-minute walk test +/− oxygen saturation NYHA functional assessment BODE index

Transplantation at a Glance, First Edition. Menna Clatworthy, Christopher Watson, Michael Allison and John Dark.

Indications for lung transplantation

Lung transplantation is indicated for end-stage obstructive, septic, restrictive lung disease or pulmonary vascular disease. In broad terms, the presence of septic disease (e.g. cystic fibrosis) or pulmonary hypertension is an indication for bilateral lung transplantation; obstructive or restrictive disease may be treated by single or bilateral lung transplantation. Combined heart–lung transplantation, popular in the 1990s, is now rarely performed, although may be indicated for some complex congenital heart diseases.

A decision to offer lung transplantation is based on physical status, quality of life and comorbidity.

Assessment investigations

Forced expiratory volume in one second (FEV₁) is the amount of breath forcibly exhaled in 1 second. It is usually expressed as a proportion of the value predicted for age, sex and build. A reduced FEV_1 signifies obstruction to air escaping.

Forced vital capacity (FVC) is the total amount of breath forcibly exhaled.

Diffusing capacity of the lung for carbon monoxide (DLCO), also called the carbon monoxide transfer factor. Carbon monoxide (CO) is avidly taken up by erythrocytes, and when inhaled, the difference between the inspired and expired partial pressure of CO reflects the ability of CO to diffuse across the alveoli, and thus reflects the alveolar surface area. It is reduced in pulmonary fibrosis.

BODE index: the body mass index, airflow obstruction, dyspnoea and exercise capacity index is a derived score that predicts mortality from chronic obstructive pulmonary disease (COPD).

Gastro-oesophageal reflux disease (GORD): severe reflux is associated with repeated aspiration and early onset obliterative bronchiolitis. Reflux is particularly common with cystic fibrosis. Patients undergo 24-hour oesophageal pH studies and barium swallow.

Bone density (DEXA) scan: osteoporosis is common in chronic respiratory disease, in part associated with chronic steroid therapy, and is associated with pathological fractures. Severe osteoporosis (T score <3.5) is a relative contraindication.

Body mass index: low BMI ($<18\,kg/m^2$) is associated with poor outcome; high BMI ($>30\,kg/m^2$) creates surgical difficulties.

Disease-specific considerations

Chronic obstructive pulmonary disease (COPD)

COPD is the most common indication for lung transplantation. Features that suggest lung transplantation may be appropriate are:

- FEV_1 <20%; DLCO <20%
- resting hypoxia (PO_2 <8 kPa) and hypercapnia (PCO_2 >6 kPa)
- pulmonary hypertension (systolic PA pressure >40 mmHg on echo).
- right-sided heart failure due to chronic pulmonary hypertension
- BODE score >7.

Cystic fibrosis (CF)

CF is characterised by periods of relative good health in the face of lungs colonised by pathogens, punctuated by severe infectious exacerbations. Transplantation is indicated in those with poor lung function (FEV_1 < 30%; FVC, 40%) or rapidly decreasing lung function and/or increasing frequency and severity of infective exacerbations. Other indications for transplantation include recurrent or refractory pneumothoraces and uncontrolled haemoptysis. Young female diabetics are at risk of early deterioration.

Patients with highly resistant organisms, particular those with *Burkholderia cenocepacia* or atypical mycobacteria (e.g. *Mycobacterium abscessus or M. kansasii*) have poor outcomes and many centres will not accept them for transplantation.

CF is a systemic disease. Diabetes is very common, and must be well controlled. Most patients have a degree of hepatic insufficiency which, if severe, may warrant combined lung–liver transplant.

Idiopathic pulmonary fibrosis (IPF)

IPF has a poor prognosis for which there is no treatment. Patients with IPF have the highest rate of death on the waiting list so early referral and transplantation is required for a successful outcome. Patients with the following should be considered:

- >10% fall in FVC in 6 months;
- DLCO <35%;
- >15% fall in DLCO in 6 months;
- resting hypoxaemia (O_2 saturations <88%) or desaturation during 6-minute walk.

Primary pulmonary hypertension

Primary pulmonary artery hypertension is associated with syncope, peripheral oedema, ascites, haemoptysis and chest pain. Patients with rapidly progressive disease, poor functional status (NYHA grade III/IV and low 6-minute walk test [<350 m]), in spite of maximal medical therapy should be considered.

Although right ventricular function is often very poor by the time of transplantation, it can improve back to normal. Combined heart and lung transplants are therefore no longer warranted.

Bronchiectasis

Similar criteria as for cystic fibrosis.

Alpha-1 anti-trypsin deficiency

Similar criteria as for COPD.

Priority for transplantation

When donor lungs become available there is often a choice between transplanting a patient with COPD who is very handicapped by their disease, albeit in a stable condition with a low waiting list mortality, and someone who is relatively well with CF but who may deteriorate and die very quickly.

At present in the UK 25% of patients awaiting a lung transplant will die in the first year on the waiting list, and only 30% will have been transplanted.

Contraindications to transplantation

There are general and specific contraindications. The general ones are similar to those mentioned for other organ transplants.

Good cardiac function, and the absence of severe coronary artery disease is important. This is especially the case for recipients with COPD, many of whom will have been heavy smokers.

CF patients are often malnourished, and a BMI of less than 18 predicts less good outcome.

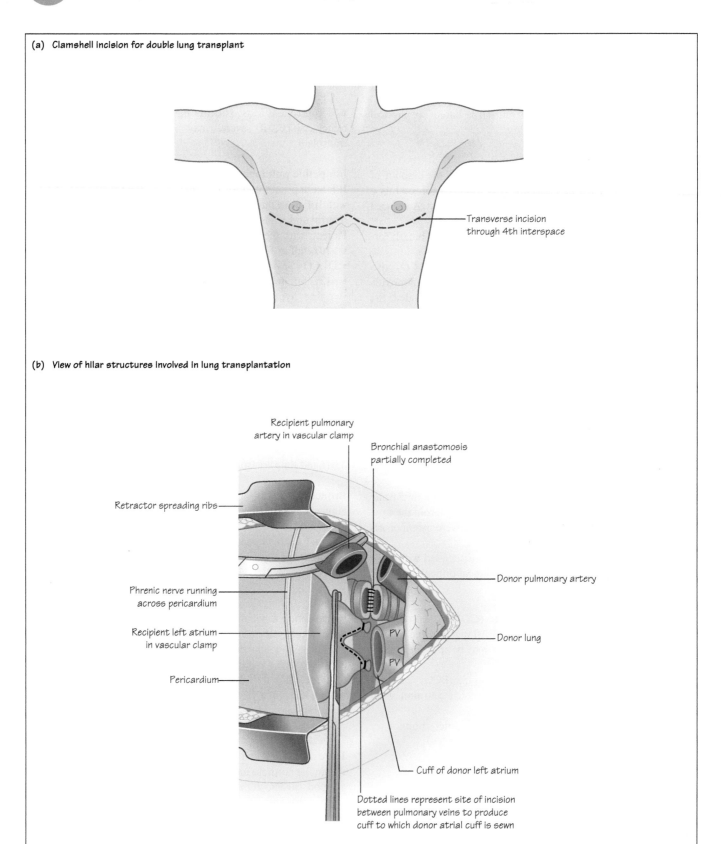

(a) Clamshell incision for double lung transplant

Transverse incision through 4th interspace

(b) View of hilar structures involved in lung transplantation

Recipient pulmonary artery in vascular clamp

Bronchial anastomosis partially completed

Retractor spreading ribs

Donor pulmonary artery

Phrenic nerve running across pericardium

Recipient left atrium in vascular clamp

PV

Donor lung

PV

Pericardium

Cuff of donor left atrium

Dotted lines represent site of incision between pulmonary veins to produce cuff to which donor atrial cuff is sewn

The lung donor

Donor selection

Matching donor and recipient involves matching blood group and donor size, and avoiding any incompatible HLA antigens that might result in hyperacute or early humoral rejection. Size is very important, particularly avoiding putting large lungs into small chests, which will result in pulmonary collapse and infection.

Lung assessment differs between DCD and DBD donors.

Lung retrieval from donors following brain death

In DBD donors, where the heart is still beating, the donor undergoes bronchoscopy before retrieval surgery commences to look for evidence of infection or inflammation; bronchial aspirates are sent for Gram stain and culture to inform choice of antibiotics in the recipient. Once the operation begins the lungs are inspected externally and care is taken to ensure that all segments are fully inflated, with no evidence of atelectasis, consolidation, masses or trauma. Pulmonary vein oxygen levels are measured by aspirating blood directly from left and right upper and lower pulmonary veins. A PO$_2$ >40 kPa is desirable.

The lungs are preserved by perfusing a low-potassium/dextran preservation solution (Perfadex), together with a prostaglandin vasodilator, via the pulmonary artery, with the lungs ventilated to aid distribution of perfusate. Following this, additional retrograde perfusion is given via the pulmonary veins to wash out clots. This may also perfuse the bronchial arteries, which arise directly from the descending thoracic aorta.

Lung donation from donors following circulatory death

Retrieving lungs from DCD donors is different. Pre-operative bronchoscopy cannot be performed. Instead, once death is confirmed the donor is re-intubated and the lungs are inflated with oxygen; at this point they are no longer ischaemic. Ideally, a nasogastric tube is placed prior to treatment withdrawal and the stomach emptied to prevent reflux of gastric contents entering the lungs at the time of death.

Increasingly lungs are being placed on an ex vivo lung perfusion (EVLP) preservation machine, which circulates preservation fluid (Steen solution) through the vessels at 37°C while the lungs are insufflated with oxygen. On this apparatus the lung can be carefully evaluated, with pulmonary venous sampling to check alveolar function and bronchoscopy. The EVLP device also permits longer storage periods and may recondition lungs, allowing previously unsuitable organs to be transplanted.

Lung transplantation

Most recipients undergo bilateral lung transplant, sometimes referred to as the sequential single lung transplant. Anastomoses of artery, bronchus and a cuff of left atrium are performed at the lung hilum. Removal of all the infected material is clearly mandatory for patients with septic lung disease. Those with pulmonary vascular disease benefit from receiving the larger vascular bed of two lungs. Patients with chronic obstructive pulmonary disease (COPD) are also best served with a bilateral lung transplant, so the single lung procedure is largely restricted to those with restrictive or fibrotic conditions.

Cardiopulmonary bypass

Traditionally, lung transplantation has been performed with the patient on cardiopulmonary bypass. This offers the advantage of haemodynamic stability as the mediastinum is being manipulated, and may allow the vascular anastomoses to be performed without clamps. The disadvantages of bypass are that it requires systemic heparinsation (which can pose significant bleeding problems if infection and inflammation has caused the lungs to adhere to the parietal pleura), renal impairment, platelet dysfunction and the use of blood products. The current trend is away from routine use of cardiopulmonary bypass. However, it is indicated if single lung ventilation causes significant hypoxia, if clamping the pulmonary artery or manipulating the mediastinum cause instability, or in patients already on extra-corporeal membrane oxygenator (ECMO) support at the time of transplant.

Single and bilateral lung transplantation

Single lung transplantation is usually performed through a posterolateral thoracotomy, particularly if cardiopulmonary bypass is not required. Bilateral lung transplantation is usually performed through a transverse incision in the fourth interspace with division of the sternum, termed a clamshell incision. This gives access to the hilar of both lungs, as well as to the heart if cardiopulmonary bypass is required. The lungs are transplanted sequentially, with the poorest functioning lung replaced first. A double-lumen endotracheal tube is placed to allow separate ventilation of each lung. In patients without pleural adhesions, there is an increasing emphasis on smaller, separate anterior thoracotomies.

The operative procedure involves dissecting the pulmonary arteries and veins free from surrounding tissue, and isolating the bronchus. Care is taken to avoid damage to the phrenic and vagal nerves. The pulmonary arteries and then the veins are ligated and divided, following which the bronchus is divided and the lung removed. In septic lung disease, such as cystic fibrosis, pneumonectomy can be a tedious and bloody affair, but good haemostasis is important, because once the new lung is in place the posterior chest wall will not be visible.

With the new lung in the hemithorax the bronchial anastomosis is completed first. Following this the pulmonary artery anastomosis is fashioned and finally a clamp is placed across the left atrium to include the origins of both pulmonary veins; these are opened as a branch patch (*see* Chapter 35) and a donor left atrial cuff is sewn to the recipient patch. The lung is then reperfused slowly. The procedure is repeated on the opposite side.

Reperfusion of the lung is performed keeping the artery pressures low (<20 mmHg). The initial blood returning from the transplanted lung to the heart is cold, full of ischaemic metabolites and may contain air, which causes embolism, particularly in the right coronary artery that lies most anterior. Myocardial instability at this stage is possible.

Post-operative analgesia is important, and a thoracic epidural should be routine after the full clamshell incision.

Heart–lung transplantation

In heart–lung transplantation the organs are transplanted as a single bloc of tissue through a median sternotomy incision. The phrenic and vagal nerves are more at risk and extra care is taken to avoid damage to them; the recurrent laryngeal nerve may also be damaged as the pulmonary artery is dissected off the aorta in the region of the ligamentum arteriosum. In patients with congenital heart disease, large collateral vessels in the mediastinum make dissection more difficult. The airway anastomosis is between donor and recipient trachea; the other anastomoses are to superior vena cava, inferior vena cava and aorta.

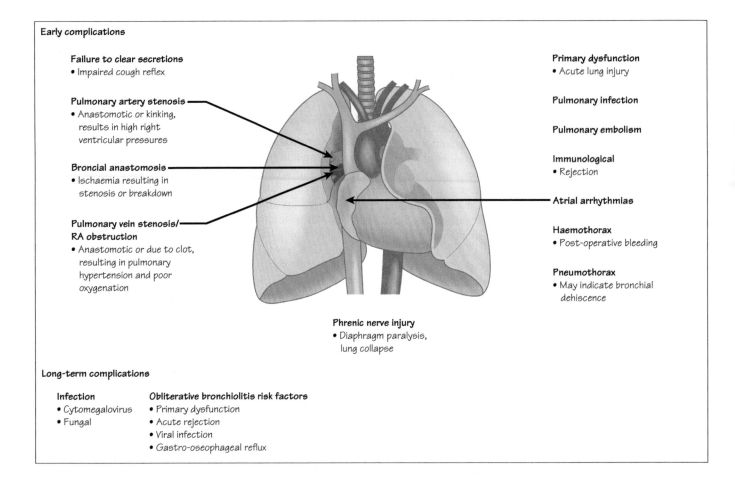

Early complications

Failure to clear secretions
• Impaired cough reflex

Pulmonary artery stenosis
• Anastomotic or kinking, results in high right ventricular pressures

Broncial anastomosis
• Ischaemia resulting in stenosis or breakdown

Pulmonary vein stenosis/ RA obstruction
• Anastomotic or due to clot, resulting in pulmonary hypertension and poor oxygenation

Primary dysfunction
• Acute lung injury

Pulmonary infection

Pulmonary embolism

Immunological
• Rejection

Atrial arrhythmias

Haemothorax
• Post-operative bleeding

Pneumothorax
• May indicate bronchial dehiscence

Phrenic nerve injury
• Diaphragm paralysis, lung collapse

Long-term complications

Infection
• Cytomegalovirus
• Fungal

Obliterative bronchiolitis risk factors
• Primary dysfunction
• Acute rejection
• Viral infection
• Gastro-oseophageal reflux

Early complications

Initial post-transplant management

The early management of patients post-lung transplantation involves limiting airway pressures (<35 mmHg) and physiotherapy to improve expectoration; tracheostomy may be indicated to facilitate tracheal toilet if prolonged intubation is anticipated. Fluid management aims to keep the recipient in a negative balance so as not to waterlog the lungs, and colloids may be preferred to crystalloids for the same reason.

Complications

The early complications following lung transplantation may be divided into four types.

1 Technical complications relating to the surgery

These are now uncommon.

• *Airway anastomosis* – the bronchial anastomosis (or tracheal if heart–lung) was the Achilles heel of the lung transplant procedure. The bronchi derive a blood supply from bronchial arteries coming directly off the thoracic aorta; these are not usually reimplanted. The donor bronchi are hence ischaemic. Anastomosis close to the lung hilum, with a very short donor bronchus, largely eliminates disruption and its catastrophic consequences.

• *Nerve injury* – the phrenic nerve is prone to damage as it runs along the pericardium near the hilar structures. The resultant diaphragmatic dysfunction may result in collapse (and then consolidation) of the lung because full expansion on inspiration cannot be achieved.

• *Pneumothorax* may result from rupture of bullae or may signify an anastomotic breakdown of the airway. Diagnosis may involve bronchoscopy to verify the integrity of the anastomosis. Most air leaks post transplant are from the lung parenchyma.

• *Haemothorax* is particular common where the lung has been infected and stuck to the parietal pleura, making removal difficult and bloody.

• *Atrial arrhythmias*, such as atrial fibrillation, are common and reflect clamping the left atrium. Most resolve spontaneously or after cardioversion.

2 Lung complications

• *Primary graft dysfunction* is the most important complication after lung transplant. It is a type of acute lung injury affecting the donor lung(s) secondary to ischaemia/reperfusion of the graft and is characterised by:

    – alveolar and interstitial peri-hilar infiltrates (representing fluid and inflammatory cells)

Transplantation at a Glance, First Edition. Menna Clatworthy, Christopher Watson, Michael Allison and John Dark.

– decreased lung compliance as the lungs become stiffer

– deteriorating gas exchange.

Prolonged ventilation is required and nitric oxide and prostaglandins have been used. Extracorporeal membrane oxygenation may be required if gas exchange is very poor.

• *Pulmonary infection* is common, and related to several factors:

– prolonged intubation and ventilation of the donor, with colonisation

– prolonged intubation of the lung transplant recipient

– prior colonisation of the lungs/trachea, especially in cystic fibrosis

– impaired mucociliary 'escalator'.

3 Extrathoracic complications

Gut complications are common and are of three sorts.

• *Delayed gastric emptying*, possibly related to vagal nerve damage; it may result in reflux and aspiration if not treated.

• *Meconium ileus equivalent*, a form of intestinal obstruction affecting patients with cystic fibrosis.

• *Acute colonic pseudo-obstruction*, which may result in colonic perforation if untreated. This particularly affects older patients with COPD.

4 Immunological complications

Acute rejection is the most common immunological complication. Occasionally in very debilitated patients, graft versus host disease may occur, where the lung has sufficient immune cells to mount an immune response against the recipient – this is also a rare complication of liver transplantation.

Late complications

Infection

Beyond the first month viral complications become more important, particularly the following two viruses.

• *Cytomegalovirus* (CMV), which can cause a severe pneumonitis in CMV-naive recipients of lungs from a donor previously infected with CMV.

• *Epstein-Barr virus*, which is associated with post-transplant lymphoma.

Fungal infections may also occur some time after transplantation, of which aspergillus is the most serious.

Bronchiolitis obliterans syndrome (BOS)

This is the manifestation of chronic allograft rejection in the lung. It is characterised by increased breathlessness, deterioration of the pulmonary function tests (FEV_1, FVC), and an obstructive picture on high-resolution computed tomography (CT) with bronchial dilatation and air trapping. Biopsy reveals obliterative bronchiolitis, where the bronchial epithelium is lost and the bronchioles are occluded by intraluminal granulation tissue. It may be a slow, insidious process, or occur rapidly following a stimulus. Risk factors include any precipitating lung injury, such as previous primary graft dysfunction, recurrent acute rejection, viral infection such as CMV, bacterial infection and gastro-oesophageal reflux disease.

Immunosuppression-related complications

As with other forms of transplant, the long-term complications of immunosuppressive drugs also affect lung transplant recipients, such as calcineurin inhibitor-induced renal impairment and diabetes.

The complications of being immunosuppressed also affect this group, with post-transplant lymphoma and other cancers being more common.

Long-term survival

More than 80% of recipients will survive the first year post transplant, and around 50% of patients will survive 10 years. The best results are in younger patients with cystic fibrosis. Retransplantation of the lung is not commonly undertaken, because there is a severe shortage of donor lungs.

(a) Schematic of full face transplant

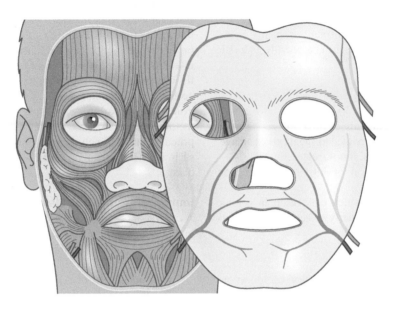

Vascularised from arterial and venous branches

Other underlying structures, such as mandible or
maxilla which may be incorporated as required

(b) Schematic of hand transplant

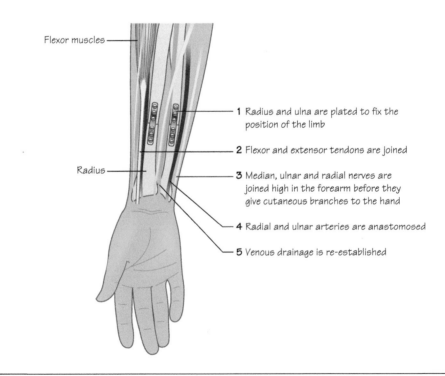

Flexor muscles

Radius

1 Radius and ulna are plated to fix the
position of the limb

2 Flexor and extensor tendons are joined

3 Median, ulnar and radial nerves are
joined high in the forearm before they
give cutaneous branches to the hand

4 Radial and ulnar arteries are anastomosed

5 Venous drainage is re-established

Transplantation at a Glance, First Edition. Menna Clatworthy, Christopher Watson, Michael Allison and John Dark.

Vascularised composite tissue allotransplantation (CTA) reflects the fact that the vascularised graft includes many different tissues, such as bone, nerve, muscle, tendons and skin. The most common example is hand transplantation, but face, laryngeal and abdominal wall transplantation are other examples. Abdominal wall transplants have been used in a few multivisceral transplant recipients to gain abdominal domain – in other words to make room for the bowel.

Hand transplantation

Indications

Loss of one hand causes significant disability and carries many psychological and social stigmata, but loss of both upper limbs is a devastating handicap. While prosthetics may provide a substitute that can be used to compensate for loss of a single limb, none can substitute for the tactile sense that is required for many activities of daily living. The benefits of such transplantation need to be balanced against the need for immunosuppression. Possible indications include:

• bilateral hand amputation;
• loss of a single upper limb but already requiring immunosuppression;
• loss of the dominant hand – this is a relative indication and the benefits need to be balanced against the risks of immunosuppression and the psychology of the recipient.

The candidates are usually trauma victims, often as a result of anti-personnel explosive devices. Transplantation is not usually considered for congenital anomalies or loss of limb due to cancer.

Assessment

Defining the requirements

It is important to define what is required by assessing the length of residual limb (hand, forearm, upper arm) and its functionality. Skin colour is also noted to try to achieve a reasonable match.

Patient evaluation

Although the surgery is long it is not as physically stressful to the recipient as other forms of transplantation. Nevertheless evaluation of cardiovascular fitness is important, as with any transplant.

Psychological assessment is very important, due to the body image issues involved. It is important to counsel recipients to manage their expectations. The first successful hand transplant was lost within 3 years due to non-compliance with medication, a consequence of the recipient's failure to come to terms with his new limb.

While functional recovery is superior to a prosthesis, and better following a single limb than a double limb transplant, it is nevertheless not perfect.

The transplant procedure

The patient is positioned with a tourniquet occluding the blood in the upper limb. The operative procedure involves the following sequence: bone fixation to existing limb bone; flexor and extensor tendon repair; nerve repair; finally the arterial and venous anastomoses are fashioned, all using microsurgical techniques. The tourniquet is then released, reperfusing the hand.

Following surgery, rehabilitation is a long process involving extensive physiotherapy. Motor and sensory recovery are good but take time as the nerves regenerate slowly; the higher the level of amputation the poorer the recovery, particularly motor recovery. Perceptive and discriminative sensation improve in hand recipients, while discriminative sensation shows less recovery in forearm recipients. The results are generally as good as can be achieved by reimplantation of someone's own hand after traumatic amputation.

Face transplantation

Face transplantation is uncommon (around 10 worldwide at the time of writing), and the term belittles the extent of what is involved. Varying components of the donor face, including lips, chin, nose, eyelids and eyebrows, may be transplanted together with the underlying tissues, possibly including the bones of the facial skeleton, such as the maxilla and mandible. The first face transplant was performed in France in 2005, and to date there have been very few such transplants, the activity being restricted as much by the lack of consent as by the psychological impact on the recipient.

Potential recipients are patients who have suffered traumatic disfigurement; the first recipient had lost her nose, mouth and chin following a dog attack; one recipient has had a transplant for plexiform neurofibromatosis; others have been victims of insults such as shotgun injuries or electrical burns. Loss of tissue due to malignancy is generally a contraindication on account of the effects of immunosuppression on the likelihood of recurrence.

As with hand transplantation the principle non-immunological issues are the psychological assessment and continued support of the recipient.

Since it is undesirable to perform repeated biopsies of the skin of the face to monitor for rejection, a separate piece of donor skin is transplanted to the arm to permit frequent biopsies; oral mucosa can also be biopsied easily if required.

The long-term outcomes of face and hand transplantation remain uncertain.

Immunosuppression and rejection

One of the principal reasons that transplantation of composite tissues has taken so long to come to the clinic was the belief that rejection would represent an insurmountable challenge. Immunosuppression for skin grafting in animals, for example, is the biggest challenge of any new immunosuppressant or tolerance-induction programme. It turns out that the immunological response to composite tissues is not as aggressive as once thought, and that it can be managed by a standard regimen of lymphocyte-depleting induction agent and tacrolimus, mycophenolate and steroid maintenance.

Rejection has been shown to occur in any of the tissues transplanted, and may be in isolation (asynchronous) or occur at the same time as rejection of other tissues (synchronous). Examples of this also exist in other organs, such that a pancreas may reject while a kidney transplanted at the same time does not, or the small bowel may reject while the colon does not.

(a) Which species?

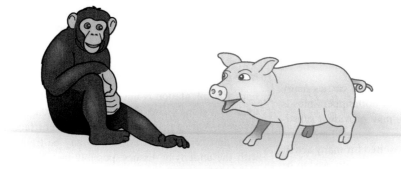

Considerations
- Ease of breeding
- Gestation period
- Animal husbandry
- Genetic manipulation
- Size of organs
- Physiology of organs

(b) Physiology

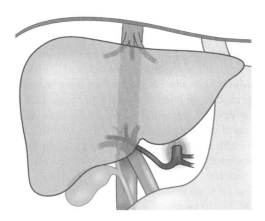

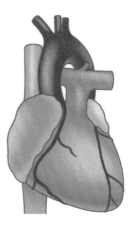

Porcine proteins differ from human
- Different concentrations
- Different structure
- Different efficacy in man

Pig BP is lower than BP in man

Pig endothelium does not regulate human clotting factors causing thrombosis

(c) Immunology

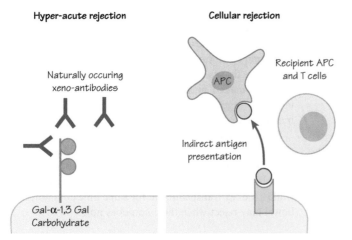

Hyper-acute rejection

Naturally occuring xeno-antibodies

Gal-α-1,3 Gal Carbohydrate

Cellular rejection

APC

Recipient APC and T cells

Indirect antigen presentation

(d) Zoonoses: PERVs

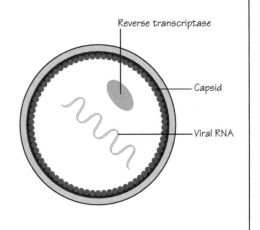

Reverse transcriptase

Capsid

Viral RNA

Transplantation at a Glance, First Edition. Menna Clatworthy, Christopher Watson, Michael Allison and John Dark.

Aspirations for xenotransplantation

The shortfall between the number of available organs for transplantation and the number of patients on the transplant waiting lists is ever widening. One solution to this that has been explored since Jaboulay's first efforts in the 1900s is the use of animal organs, so-called xenotransplantation. In spite of much research, xenotransplantation has failed to achieve the successes hoped for, and with every new finding more hurdles appear to slow its progress.

Many xenotransplants have been performed, ranging from kidney, liver and heart transplants using dog, goat, pig or primate organs, to the transplantation of specialised cells in an attempt to cure diabetes or Parkinson's disease. None has yet been successful.

Barriers to success

Donor selection

It is generally agreed that the favoured animal for mass breeding as donors for transplantation is the pig, for the following reasons.

• The animals are of a similar size to man, compared with primates such as baboons, which are much smaller.
• Organs are anatomically similar to those in man.
• Breeding programmes are well established, and gestation is short.
• Genetic manipulation has been shown to be possible.

In the paragraphs that follow we have assumed that the pig is the donor; similar considerations apply whatever the species chosen.

Physiology

There are several physiological considerations to xenotransplantation.

1 *Environmental differences.* There are several differences in the environment in which organs exist in pig and man.
  • Temperature: the core temperature of a pig is 2°C higher than man at 39°C.
  • Blood pressure: the pig's blood pressure is lower than that of a human. Will a pig heart be able to support an effective blood pressure in man? Similarly, what will be the effect of a normal human blood pressure on pig organs such as the kidney?

2 *Protein differences.* There are subtle differences in structure and efficacy of some pig proteins compared with man. For example some of the clotting factors (e.g. factor V) exist in far higher concentrations in pig than man, the significance of which is not clear. Among the vast number of metabolic processes and proteins that are produced by the liver it is unlikely that all will be compatible with man, which makes liver transplantation from pig to man the least likely xenotransplant to succeed.

3 *Regulatory proteins* exist on endothelium to prevent inappropriate activation of protective mechanisms such as complement and coagulation. Pig liver produces pig complement, but the proteins involved in regulating human complement do not have the same regulatory effect on pig complement. Similarly the regulatory proteins on pig endothelium that stop clot forming are not effective against primate coagulation factors, so thrombosis is a common

experimental finding when transplanting pig hearts into primates.

4 *Hormone differences.* While some pig hormones are known to be efficacious in man, such as insulin, it is not clear whether human hormones will have the same effect on pig organs, and whether the same degree of regulation of hormone secretion will occur.

5 *Longevity.* Most animals have a shorter life span than man. Will organs from pigs be able to support life for as long as a human organ, or will they suffer changes of senescence more quickly?

Immunology

Humoral response: natural antibodies

Man posses natural antibodies to a carbohydrate residue on pig cells known as Gal-α-1,3 Gal, which is produced by the enzyme α-galactosyl transferase. This is present in many mammals but not New World primates or man. These pre-formed natural antibodies (XNAbs) cause hyperacute rejection, a process that involves the XNAbs binding to the porcine cells and fixing complement. XNAbs arise as a consequence of an immune response to enteric bacteria that contain the same residues; the XNAbs are absent at birth but appear soon after.

Strategies to overcome XNAb-mediated hyperacute rejection
Genetic manipulation of pigs has resulted in strains that bear human complement regulatory proteins on the cell surface (DAF, MCP and CD59). These proteins protect the cells from attack by human complement, even after the XNAbs have bound. More recently strains have been developed that do not express Gal-α-1,3 Gal ('Gal knockout' pigs). Neither strategy seems to abolish completely a humoral response against the xenograft.

Cellular rejection

The major histocompatibility complex of the pig is different to that of man, and as such it was thought this would favour transplantation across species since xenorecognition of the pig proteins on pig MHC molecules would not be possible. It turns out that xenorecognition occurs via the indirect pathway, with pig proteins presented to human T cells on human antigen-presenting cells, and effector T cells are active against pig cells. Moreover, there is also a significant innate immune response against the xeno-antigens.

Zoonoses: endogenous retroviruses

A zoonosis is the transmission of an infectious agent from one species to another. One such example is believed to be the human immunodeficiency virus, a retrovirus that was originally found in primates in Africa. Research has shown that, as with other mammalian species, there are many different endogenous retroviruses in the pig genome (PERVs), the significance of which is unclear, but some have been shown to be capable of infecting human cells in culture. However, in the few cases where humans have had pig tissue implanted in the past, such as porcine skin to cover burns, there is no evidence of viral transmission to date.

Ethics

There are many ethical and religious views that would oppose breeding fellow creatures in order to sacrifice them for spare parts.

Index

Transplantation at a Glance, First Edition. Menna Clatworthy, Christopher Watson, Michael Allison and John Dark.